The Battle For Health Is Over <u>pH</u>

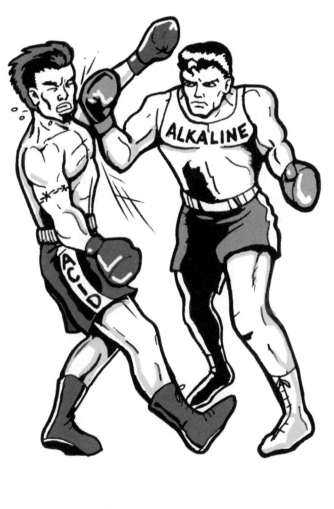

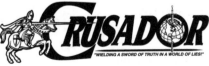

"WIELDING A SWORD OF TRUTH IN A WORLD OF LIES!"

This book is not intended to provide medical advice or to take the place of medical advice and treatment from your personal physician. This book is published for the express purpose of sharing educational information, scientific research, and biblical truth gathered from the research, studies, and experiences of the author and the health care professionals, scientists, nutritionists, and health freedom advocates who contributed their time and input to this book. Readers are advised to consult their own doctors or other qualified health care professionals regarding the treatment of their medical problems. If readers are taking prescription medications, they should consult with their physicians and not take themselves off of medicines to start supplementation without the proper supervision of a physician. Should you choose to make use of the information contained herein without first consulting a health care professional, you are prescribing for yourself, which is your Constitutional and Divine right. However, neither the author, nor the publisher assumes any responsibility for possible consequences from any treatment, action or preparation to any person reading or following the information in this book.

ISBN: 0-9720636-1-7

Copyright © 2007 by Crusador Enterprises

Address all correspondences to:
Crusador Enterprises
P.O. Box 618205
Orlando, FL 32861-8205
1-407-290-1932
www.HealthTruthRevealed.com

Printed in the United States of America

ACKNOWLEDGMENTS

"As a sports medicine physician and trainer for amateur, Olympic, and professional athletes, I have been interested in the subject of pH and how it affects my patients for quite some time. I usually find that when my athletes are running acidic they don't perform as well, they are much more susceptible to injury, they are more fatigued, and their recovery time from training takes much longer. By working with these athletes to correct imbalances, many of them report back to me that their performance is noticeably better, they have less pain during and after workouts, less injuries, and they recover much faster. When I read **The Battle For Health Is Over pH** I was relieved to finally see an articulate and powerful presentation put together on this subject. I firmly believe that pH is one area of medical science that offers much promise for athletes looking for better performance and for the general public seeking viable, science based alternatives that work in harmony with the body."

Dr. John Russell, Physician for 1988 and 1992 Olympic Track Teams – Medical Director, Florida Governor's Council for Physical Fitness and Sports – Director P.E.A.K. Performance Center

"It is so vitally important for the body to maintain proper blood pH that the body will even rob from its own oxygen, and then calcium, and then on down the line from every place else, in order to neutralize and buffer the waste and dietary acids. When people put a sufficient quantity of Active Oxygen Therapies and supplements into their bodies - for as many days as are necessary in each case - and of course that includes eating well, exercising, etc., we find the majority of people return to being perfectly healthy. At the same time their overall pH goes back to normal, slightly alkaline. This is the proof pH is a great indicator of the overall body state of readiness for health.

"By showing the prime importance and details of pH from a 'whole systems' viewpoint, **The Battle For Health Is Over pH,** makes it easy for anyone to understand how all this works, and brings all the facts together into one work so we can eliminate the common misunderstandings. Our bodies are amazingly simple (good in, equals good out) and yet at the same time very complex (try studying intercellular chemistry). This book makes it easy for you to get the information needed to win the battle for health by knowing the HOW and WHY of pH."

Ed McCabe, "Mr. Oxygen"
Bestselling author of Flood Your Body With Oxygen

Table Of Contents

FOREWORD

There have been cures for disease since the beginning of time. You just have to know where to look. The problem lies in that if it is made by God (natural), you cannot patent it, therefore there is no MONEY to be made. There is no such thing as a so-called incurable disease.

It has been my good fortune to work with and read the manuscript of a book written by my good friend Gary Tunsky, discussing the travesties of the American Medical Industry. Not only does his book address what is wrong with the current Medical System, but it also offers education and solutions as to how to implement and enjoy true health. It is so easy to point out what is wrong with an institution, but real progress is made by offering solutions.

I find it extremely important that the facts in this book be made available to the general public. It is time for those of us who have experienced the proven results of implementing treatments, as those suggested by Tunsky, to speak out and offer these natural medicines to the American public. A large majority of the population is not aware of the health solutions that this book describes and it is only by getting these facts out that we can hope to see knowledge take hold and people's thinking about health-related problems change.

I have worked with Tunsky in teaching and implementing many of the treatments that he offers in his book **"The Battle For Health Is Over pH."**

I have seen these treatments work and watched as people regained their health from seemingly untreatable disease. Tunsky has done a great job in presenting facts that have been "swept under the rug" for far too long. People must know that they do have a choice in their healthcare, that there are options and treatments that will help them to achieve health without toxic drugs and their side-effects, and most importantly, that they are <u>responsible</u> for their own health or lack of it.

Natural medicine is flourishing and people are beginning to experience the wisdom in getting to the root of an illness...not just treating the symptoms.

I hope that many who read this book will pass it along to friends, relatives, and yes, even their medical doctors. I hope that it will be read and used by all Natural Healthcare Providers as a textbook in teaching their patients the true value and meaning of being healthy.

Dr. Edward F. Group, III, D.C., Ph. D, N.D., DACBN
Founder/CEO, Global Healing Center, Inc., Houston, Texas.

"If people let the government decide what foods they eat and what medicines they take, their bodies will soon be in as sorry a state as are the souls of those who live under tyranny."

— Thomas Jefferson

"The doctor of the future will give little medicine, but will interest his patients in the care of the human frame, diet, and in the cause and prevention of disease."

— Thomas A. Edison

PART I

The Battle For Health Is Over pH

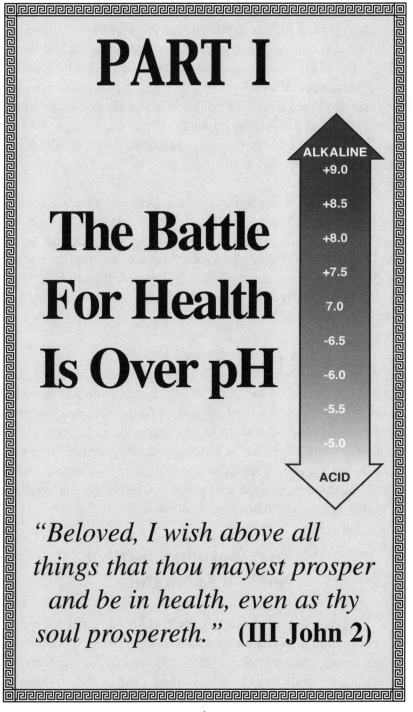

ALKALINE
+9.0
+8.5
+8.0
+7.5
7.0
-6.5
-6.0
-5.5
-5.0
ACID

"Beloved, I wish above all things that thou mayest prosper and be in health, even as thy soul prospereth." **(III John 2)**

In my twenty years of cumulative research in disease epidemiology, I have uncovered the hidden culprit lurking behind all health-related issues. Most doctors are practicing in the dark, since many of these maladies commonly elude medical diagnosis as psychosomatic or stress-related illnesses. Every human being, each one of us, regardless of our state of health, possesses some degree of acid/alkaline biochemical imbalance, because of the body's constant fight to maintain homeostasis or equilibrium. There are no exceptions to this rule.

This book is a practical guide to help you understand how effectively regulating your pH can produce lasting changes in your health. The subject of pH is definitely a complex one; however, this book will give the average person a complete understanding of pH from start to finish. In it you will learn how your body works at the cellular level, what is necessary to produce life in healthy cells, and how pH ties into the whole life process.

The percentage of Americans suffering with poor health has risen dramatically during the last fifty years. Much of this unnecessary misery is the result of our change from a time when we lived closer to nature and consumed pure, organically grown, unadulterated foods that were highly nutritious and alkalizing to the body. Today, most of us live in concrete jungles, far away from the source of real food, consuming an overwhelming quantity of unnatural, packaged, and processed foods that are synthetic, highly acidic, and damaging to our bodies.

We Were Born in a Garden, Not in a Laboratory

To enjoy optimum health, the body needs balanced quantities of natural acid and alkaline substances coming ideally from living, whole food complexes that support life. The concept of regulating the body's pH to stay well in a world full of sickness and disease is leading to a paradigm shift in nutritional science. This proven science within the field of microbiology dates back to the late 1800s. After a century of suppression by the pharmaceutical elite, it has recently become one of the hottest new trends in the health and nutrition industry.

A renowned 19th century French microbiologist named Antoine Béchamp pioneered this science-based health research. Other 20th century cellular terrain specialists such as Claude Bernard, Virginia Livingston-Wheeler, Günther Enderlein, Gaston Naessens, and Arthur Kendall advanced his research further. Their cutting-edge discoveries showed conclusive proof of the correlation between proper acid-alkaline pH balance of the body's cells, tissues, and fluids and an optimum state of health. Béchamp and his colleagues concluded that the cause of disease is not germs themselves, but rather the inner condition of the patient's cellular terrain at the time of exposure. Whether germs or pathogens incubate or remain dormant all depends upon proper cell environment and pH. Cell synthesis, hormone production, metabolic rate, neurotransmitter release, and DNA function are all signaled by the cellular pH environment, either to promote health and vitality or to promote disease.

The scientific community's adoption of Louis Pasteur's Germ Theory Of Disease as the whole truth (that germs and pathogens are the direct cause of most disease) without regard to the revelations of Antoine Béchamp's microzymian principle (that the acidic condition of the patient's cellular environment creates disease) marks one of the most controversial turns of events in modern history.

I intend to prove, beyond a shadow of a doubt, that modern, orthodox microbial medicine is based upon and illegitimately grew from fundamental scientific error, fueled by a "kill mode" mindset: i.e. **Kill the bacteria, kill the virus, kill the fungus and kill the tumor – resulting in the slow killing of the patient.**

This mindset has played a major role in the promotion of illness today by creating resistant strains of bacteria and suppressing the symptoms of illness, while leaving the illness, itself, intact.

Béchamp and these cellular terrain specialists concluded that, just as a slight variation in body temperature from 98.6 degrees can make you sick, a slight variance in the body's delicate pH balance will throw your whole system out of balance causing disease. This simple deviation of pH negatively impacts your health, setting up a cellular environment for disease in which pathogens can thrive. One of the leading indications of a health problem is when your pH level moves toward the acidic side below a neutral pH of 7.0.

What In The Cell Is Going On?

To fully understand the importance of pH regulation and how slight imbalances can lead to degenerative and metabolic disease processes, you must first become familiar with the miniature world of the cell. **All life begins in the cell, is maintained by the cell, and ceases by the cell.** As you quietly read these words, a whirl of activity is taking place in every cell of your body. Every second, millions of unseen, unnoticed new cells are reborn in your body's ceaseless program of self-regeneration.

Cells are the bricks and mortar from which all living tissues and organs are made. Each cell performs baffling chemical transformations, processing and producing an infinite number of vital, complex building materi-

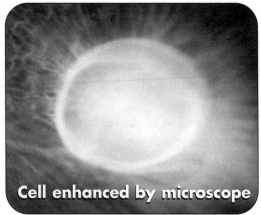

Cell enhanced by microscope

als, including vitamins, hormones, neurotransmitters, and growth factors, to protein-based peptides, neuro-peptides and enzymes, all the way through to the tiny packets of metabolic life-force energy we call adenosinetriphosphate (ATP), required to support life.

A healthy body is determined by the collective health of each one of its cells. All disease originates at the molecular and cellular level – not at the organ or system level – as we're led to believe by Western medicine. The healthy molecular building materials of oxygen, carbon, hydrogen, and nitrogen create healthy cells. Healthy cells create healthy tissues. Healthy tissues create healthy organs like the heart and lungs. Healthy organs create healthy systems like the endocrine system and the immune system. Finally, healthy body systems make up a healthy organism.

In the complex world of over 100 trillion cells that make up your body's "nation," you are the President (the brain) that delegates the police force (immune system) to protect and shield the cellular citizens from attack by foreign enemies (free radicals). The cellular citizens' habitat, their work performance, transportation system, medical care, communication, food and water, toxic waste and trash removal, are all under your control. When you

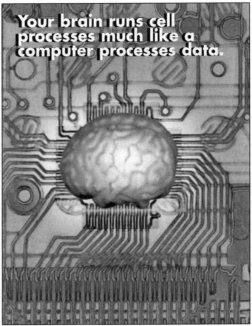

Your brain runs cell processes much like a computer processes data.

continuously eat cell nourishing foods, drink clean water, and breathe pure, clean air, your body's nation will receive all it needs for proper functioning as a whole community.

Your cell citizens come in all shapes and sizes, and perform an infinite variety of job tasks. Some reside in large cities that are your organs. Others prefer to live in the outskirts, in small towns away from the traffic, for instance, your fingernails. But no matter where they reside, each cellular citizen has a purpose, an important duty for the good of the nation – the health and maintenance of your body.

Cell Composition

There are close to 200 different types of cells that make up the architecture of the human body. There are skin cells, blood cells, nerve cells, bone, brain, and muscle cells, hair, kidney, and heart cells, liver cells, spleen cells, stem cells, eye cells, etc. They all perform unique functions that synergistically orchestrate the body's functional capacity as a whole.

Each one of these cells is a unique piece of the body puzzle that makes up the big picture. As examples, nerve cells produce neurotransmitters such as norepenephrine, serotonin, acetycholine, and dopamine for communication through nerve transmission. Skin cells produce melanin, a pigmented cell that turns the skin tan for protection against UV sunlight. Muscle cells produce adenosinetriphosphate (ATP) energy for muscle contraction. Liver cells produce HDL cholesterol and bile for fat metabolism. Beta cells in the pancreas produce insulin for blood sugar regulation. Glandular cells synthesize hormones like thyroxine, testosterone and estrogen.

Each of these cells code for a different half-life of survival, constantly dying and replacing themselves throughout your whole life span. For instance, your red blood cells die and replace themselves every 90 days. Your dermis skin layer sheds like a snake and is replaced every 21 to 28 days. You generate a whole new heart about every 8 months. You synthesize a whole new liver every 5 months. The surface layer of the mucosal lining in your intestines quickly replaces itself every 3 to 5 days. Your taste buds turn over every 10 days. Because skeletal bone cells are made up of a harder matrix of calcium, boron, osteoclasts and vitamin D, it can take up to 7-10 years for bone cells to die and replace. So everyone reading this book gets a whole new body every 7-10 years. Now, I said a new one - not a healthier one!

The new cell generations are completely dependent on the building materials you fed the previous cells, whether they were toxins or nutrients. If you were bathing the previous cells in poisons from toxic emotions and toxic food, air, water, and drugs, the next cell generation will be weaker than the one before. Future cell generations will continue to degenerate unless detoxification measures are implemented. On the other hand, if the previous cells were nurtured in water, full-spectrum nutrients, and high oxygen saturation, the next cell generation will be stronger than the original. The whole body will be progressing to a regenerative state instead of a degenerative state. Our body's cells constantly self-regulate, self-repair and self-renew under the right conditions. God has programmed them for life, not sickness and death.

What Constitutes A Healthy Cell?

There are 90-plus nutrients in ten different categories that are necessary to produce the hormones, peptides, neurotransmitters, growth factors, and other materials needed for new cell growth and proper functioning of the body systems as a whole. They are:

1. **24 amino acids**
2. **Carbohydrates or glycogen**
3. **Essential Fatty Acids**

4. **16 vitamins**
5. **72 minerals**
6. **Enzymes**
7. **Phyto-nutrients (pro-oxidants from plants)**
8. **Sunshine**
9. **Oxygen**
10. **Water**

These 90-plus nutrients are synonymous with the 26 letters of the alphabet that make up the dictionary. If you remove just 5 letters from the alphabet, you can only compile half a dictionary. Similarly, if the cells are bathed in 45 nutrients instead of the necessary 90, the cells' manufacturing potential is cut in half. This limits energy production, hormonal production, and neurotransmitter production, which then limits the peak performance of the whole body. This is analogous to a high-performance sports car's eight-cylinder engine sputtering along on only four cylinders.

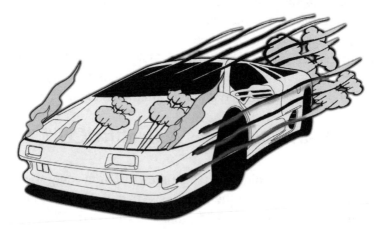

So, if the health of the cell is the answer, what constitutes a healthy cell? It all depends on the cell environment created by what you eat, drink, breathe and bathe in. You either nourish your 100 trillion cells with oxygen, water, vitamins, minerals, enzymes, phytonutrients, sunlight, essential fatty acids, glucose and amino acids, or contaminate them with man-made synthetic chemicals that slowly poison the bloodstream. What you breathe, whether it's oxygen or environmental contaminants, ends up in the bloodstream. Whatever you ingest – living, organic fruits, vegetables, nuts, grains, legumes and seeds, or refined, processed lifeless foods and toxic, sugar-laden drinks, all ends up in the bloodstream after digestion. Whatever you bathe in, tap water, toxic soaps, toxic shampoos or biodegradable organic soaps and shampoos – is absorbed through the skin and also ends up in your bloodstream.

If circulating properly, the bloodstream is a flowing river of life to all the cells, bringing nourishment and removing acidic waste residues. Picture a vibrant, gushing river that branches into streams, with streams that diverge into trickling brooks, nourishing the trees, flowers, and ambient vegetation along the way. Now picture your gushing arteries branching into veins that become trickling capillaries, nourishing your cells with nutrients and life-giving blood while picking up the trash en route. So, the question to contemplate: Is your bloodstream a flowing river of life, or a stagnant, toxic swamp of death and disease?

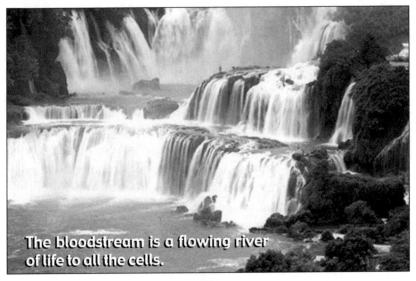

The bloodstream is a flowing river of life to all the cells.

Cells Perform Many Functions

Cells are multi-faceted. Some act as miniature electrical generators or lithium batteries, synthesizing energy (ATP), harnessing micro-voltage. All cells breathe by respiration, just like your lungs, in order to bring in oxygen and intelligent nutrients and remove toxic waste products. Cells are also manufacturing plants that synthesize hormones, neurotransmitters, proteins and life force to run bodily functions. In many ways, our cells are analogous to us as a body organism, but on a micro-scale. We communicate, cells communicate. We breathe oxygen, cells breathe oxygen. We need photon light and electromagnetic energy, cells need photon light and electromagnetic energy.

Bodily processes are so much more complicated than nutritionists and medical science have ever contemplated. Our finite minds could not possibly fathom or consciously control the extraordinarily complex tasks of manufacturing, storage, repair, communication, transportation, policing, waste disposal, administration, food production, temperature control and pH balancing that occur in our body's cells to maintain health and vitality every second of the day.

Language of the Cells

Just as people communicate in different languages using sound vibrations to create verbal language, cells communicate with each other 24-hours a day through an intricate network of electrical, magnetic, chemical, and hormonal language. The coils of the DNA helix act as transmitters and receivers of cellular information through photon emissions in the form of electromagnetic pulse wave energy. These impulses are sent to neighboring and distant cells, similar to the way a radio antenna receives and transmits sound frequency. For example, in a nerve cell the language is neuro-chemical, communicated through neurotransmitters such as dopamine, serotonin, and acetylcholine. In a muscle cell, the language is chemical, communicated through adenosinetriphosphate (ATP), produced by the mitochondria. In a glandular cell, the language is hormonal, communicated through hormones such as estrogen, adrenaline, testosterone, DHEA and cortisone, produced by the endocrine glands.

Here is an analogy of how all the cells communicate harmoniously. Envision all six billion-plus people on this planet picking up a wireless phone at the same time and having a simultaneous phone conversation. Now picture everyone clicking over to three-way and having conversations with two other people in different places throughout the world at the same time. Next, picture everyone in the world switching to a conference call with a total conversation capability of 1,000 different people talking simultaneously. This is but a fraction of what goes on every nanosecond with cellular processes. Your intestinal "cell phones" talk to the skin. Your spleen "cell phones" talk to the thymus. Your heart "cell phones" talk to the liver.

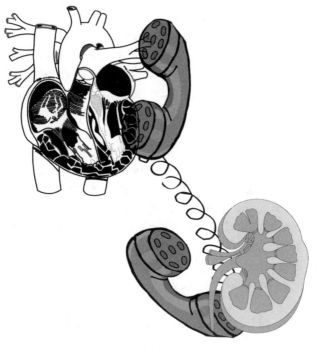

No cell, organ or system works alone, just as no nutrient works alone. They all work in unison like an orchestrated symphony. The question is, do your body's "cell phones" have good reception to transmit and receive messages freely from neighboring cells, or do they have a bad connection, due to built-up toxins around the cell membrane and DNA damage from harmful free radicals? So, just what is the regulatory authority that controls all these cell processes and ensures proper cellular communication? The answer is pH.

The Link Between pH And Cell Health

The abbreviation pH stands for the power of hydrogen. A pH test using a piece of litmus paper actually measures the concentration of positively-charged hydrogen ions in your body. Ions are electrically-charged atoms or groups of atoms that together make up the electrical "juice" or current your body uses to communicate. The more positively-charged hydrogen ions present, the more acidity is present. The fewer hydrogen ions present, the less acidity. The total pH scale ranges from one to fourteen (1-14), with seven considered to be neutral. Anything below seven is considered acidic and anything above seven is considered alkaline. Like a thermometer that measures body temperature, the pH scale shows increases and decreases in the acid/alkaline content of your body's fluids such as blood, saliva, and urine.

A healthy body functions best when it is slightly alkaline. Deviations in the blood above or below a pH range of 7.30 to 7.45 can signal potentially serious and dangerous symptoms or states of "dis-ease" which warn us of a deeper-rooted disease process. When your cell and tissue pH levels deviate from a healthy range (7.2-7.5) into an acidic state (below 7.0 pH), the acid wastes normally discarded through the body's elimination routes start to back up, as in a clogged sewage system.

The pH of your blood, tissues, and bodily fluids affects

the state of your cellular health and internal cleanliness. When your pH levels are in proper balance, you will experience a high degree of health and well-being. You will be able to resist states of "dis-ease" and the onset of chronic symptoms. Every metabolic and organ/system function depends entirely on your delicately-balanced pH, including all regulatory mechanisms such as digestion, metabolism, respiration, hormone release, neurotransmitter release, and immunity.

It is important to understand that the pH of your blood is critical to your life, to your very survival. The pH of blood has a very small degree of tolerance for variation. Your body does everything in its power to keep the pH of your blood within this neutral range, between 7.30 and 7.45, including pulling alkalizing minerals such as calcium out your bones and other body stores, if necessary.

If the body is overwhelmed by excess acids from poor diet or over-exposure to chemical and environmental toxins, built-in compensating mechanisms go into effect in an attempt to neutralize and excrete acidic toxins from the blood, cells, lymph, and tissue fluids. There are eight internal buffering systems the body uses to neutralize acids and balance pH. If these eight neutralizing mechanisms become overwhelmed and cannot function adequately, the excess acids will severely compromise cellular integrity and function, eventually causing a complete metabolic and system breakdown where serious health problems like cancer can manifest.

The Eight Built-In Acid Buffering Systems

1. Increasing Oxygenation: The most potent and effective acid-buffering compound is oxygen. The first thing the body does in an attempt to help neutralize excess toxic acid is to bring in more oxygen by increasing respiration. Increased respiration hastens the release of CO_2 from the lungs, helping to expel the gases.

According to one of the world's foremost authorities on the healing powers of oxygen, Ed McCabe, quoted here in an interview in the June-July 2004 issue of *CRUSADOR Magazine*: *"Everything that's a human waste product or a toxin that ends up in our bodies must be combined with oxygen before it can leave the body. There are four major chemical elements that combine with oxygen: sulfur, nitrogen, carbon, and hydrogen. For example, if the body wants to get rid of hydrogen, it combines it with oxygen to form water and we urinate it out. If the body wants to get rid of sulfur, it combines it with oxygen and we defecate it out. If it wants to get rid of carbon monoxide, the poisonous gas that's a result of respiration – a waste product, it adds oxygen to it, makes it into CO2 or carbon dioxide, and we breathe it out. <u>All the waste products within the human body must have oxygen combined with them or they can't leave (including all acids)."* (1)

2. Utilizing Amino Acid Reserves: The second step the body undertakes to buffer or neutralize acids is to grab intra-cellular amino acids, such as cysteine, taurine, glutathione and methionine, from protein digestion and pull them into the blood. These alkalizing amino acids work to bind acids for removal through the skin by sweating or through the kidneys by urination. This is why it is important to consume high-quality proteins in your diet. Bio-available, amino acid-rich protein foods such as organically-raised free-range turkey, salmon, cold water fish, organic eggs, nuts, seeds, beans, ionized whey protein, or crystalline, free-form amino acid supplements taken on a regular basis, all serve to assure adequate amino acids to help pH regulation.

3. Utilizing High pH Body Fluids: Next in line are high-pH body fluids such as lymph and saliva, which work like a solvent to dilute and neutralize acid residues. This is why it is extremely important to keep the body properly hydrated. Water is a solvent. Over 90% of the population is dehydrated from an over-consumption of acidic, dehydrating foods and beverages including coffee, alcohol, carbonated drinks and high-sodium fast food. If the body is not properly hydrated, fluid reserves from the blood, saliva and lymph are depleted, thus limiting their acid neutralizing properties.

4. Pulling High pH Electrolytes from Bones, Teeth, and Muscles: The fourth adaptation response for neutralizing acids is to pull alkaline electrolytes such as calcium, magnesium, potassium, sodium, and vital trace minerals from the bones, teeth and muscles. These minerals bind to acid salts from intra-cellular and extra-cellular fluids where they are excreted through the kidneys/bladder as urine waste.

It is absolutely imperative that adequate ionic or plant-based minerals are taken in through diet or supplementation to replenish the body's alkaline mineral reserves. Otherwise, the eventual result is severe mineral deficiency, further escalating the progression of disease.

5. Filtering Acids through The Body's Elimination Routes: The fifth bodily response to disperse excess acids is excretion through the filtration and elimination systems of the skin, urinary tract, colon, and respiratory system. When these systems become overwhelmed and congested, excess acids build up in weak tissues, organs, and cells. If not corrected, this can lead to a serious, spiraling acidic condition.

Any truly effective pH restoration program must focus on: **A.)** Opening the skin pores through sweat (diaphoresis) to assist the body in eliminating acids **B.)** Drinking plenty of mineralized, high pH water to hydrate the body and flush out excess acids **C.)** Cleansing the colon to eliminate stagnant acidic wastes **D.)** Increasing respiration to release CO2 and bring in more oxygen to bind acids and pull them out of the body **E.)** Purifying the liver and kidneys to filter acids from the blood.

6. **Manufacturing High pH Bicarbonate Ions:** If the previous five systems cannot eliminate acids quickly enough, the body will compensate by manufacturing high pH bicarbonate ions from CO_2, diffusing them into the blood plasma to perform this neutralization. This is why it is very important to support the first five systems, to prevent the body from entering into the disease conditions described in #7 and #8.

7. **Pushing Excess Acids to Outer Extremities:** If these first six adaptation responses do not properly eliminate the acids, the body's last ditch attempt will be to push the excess acids and toxins into outer extremities as a storage bin away from vital organs. These low-priority storage deposition areas happen to be places in the body where disease symptoms of pain and inflammation are most often felt. Examples are: acid residues that are stored in the wrists (carpel tunnel syndrome), in the knees (osteoarthritis), in the feet and toes (gout), in the skin (dermatitis and eczema), in the joints and fingers (rheumatoid arthritis), and in the tissues (fibromyalgia, chronic fatigue and other degenerative diseases).

8. **Dumping Acids into The Blood and Vital Organs:** Once these non-vital storage deposits are filled, the last adaptive response will be to deposit the excess acids into the blood, which then transfer into the vital organs through circulation. At this late stage, the body will more than likely be manifesting serious disease conditions such as blood disorders, cancer, diabetes, heart disease, debilitating arthritis, and/or a host of other chronic degenerative diseases. Following the advice I recommend in the first five stages and my **7-7-7 Program of Perfect Health** (listed at the end of this book) is critical to removing stagnant acid wastes or deposits in the blood before they get delivered to the cells.

If all these built-in buffering systems are overwhelmed, the end result is an accumulated toxic load that destroys cells and damages DNA. It overloads the filtration systems, the elimination routes, cells, and immune system, leading to degenerative disease and premature death. These intelligent compensatory systems are what keep you alive.

The path of least resistance is to transfer the toxins from the bloodstream to your weakest organ in the chain of organs for storage. The targeted organ for the deposition of acid residues correlates with the descriptive label of cellular malfunction placed by medical science. If the acid storage is around the pancreatic beta cells that produce insulin, the fancy disease label is diabetes mellitus. If acid toxins accumulate in the colon, you will exhibit the symptoms of what is called diverticulitis, Crohn's Disease, leaky gut, dysbiosis, constipation or colon cancer; take your pick. If acid toxins accumulate around the myelin sheathing of the nerves, the name will be Multiple Sclerosis (MS) or ALS (Lou Gehrig's disease). If they accumulate around the nerve fibers, it's Guillain-Barré or myasthenia gravis. If the acids accumulate around the substantia nigra (dopamine-producing cells), it's called Parkinson's disease. The medical mystery labels go on and on.

To assist the burden of the eight internal buffering systems that automatically kick in to balance pH, any true restoration program should incorporate the following five protocols:

1) Increase oxygen through ozone therapy, oxygen drops, hyperbaric chamber, deep breathing techniques, etc.
2) Increase blood circulation through exercise, lymph massage, light beam generator, low-level laser, and/or Chi machine.
3) Eliminate acid toxins by doing a complete detoxification program starting with colon, then liver, kidneys, lymph, and blood.
4) Eliminate all synthetic, manmade acids from the diet, especially all sources of refined, processed sugar.
5) Consume large amounts of alkaline green foods and fresh

vegetable juices rich in chlorophyll (wheat grass, barley grass, alfalfa grass, kamut grass, spirulina, chlorella, etc.) along with alkalizing minerals, water, and phytonutrients.

The Cascading Cycle of Acid pH

The primary cause of the cascading cycle of acid pH is oxygen deprivation. Nothing impedes or hinders the body's assimilation of oxygen more than acid. In fact, oxygen deficiency or hypoxia is the major culprit in today's epidemic of acid-related diseases. Only ample supplies of oxygen and vital minerals will guarantee that your cells "breathe" adequately and balance your pH levels.

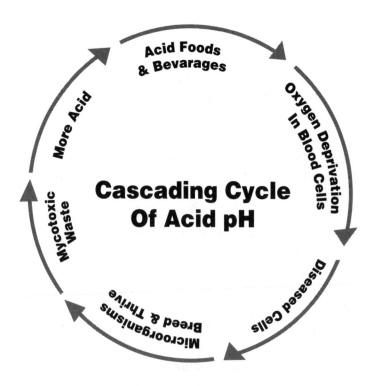

There are five main factors that contribute to the body's oxygen deficit.

A.) Lowered atmospheric oxygen caused by environmental contaminants. There have been over 100,000 environmental pollutants dumped into our air over the last 50 years, reducing atmospheric oxygen levels in some major industrial cities from 21.9% to below 17%. At 7%, life as we know it ceases to exist.
B.) Pollution of oceans, lakes, and rivers, destroying the oxygen-producing plankton and algae.
C.) Destruction of the rain forest, which contributes significantly to the earth's oxygen demise.
D.) Low oxygen saturation of the blood due to shallow breathing and sedentary lifestyles.
E.) Poor dietary habits that overwhelm the body with toxins and acids and interfere with cellular respiration.

Fundamentally, all regulatory systems from breathing, digestion, circulation, hormone production, and neurotransmitter release, serve the purpose of balancing pH by removing the acids normally generated by body tissues and cells.

When the cellular matrix that makes up the tissues and organs is suffocated, the cells cannot breathe properly or receive the nutrient building blocks they need for manufacturing tasks. Acidic pH, coupled with a lack of circulation from a sedentary lifestyle, results in stagnant extra-cellular waste. Once the cell membranes become coated and solidified by acid poisons, the cells begin to spill out CO_2 and lactic acid wastes, adding to an already acidic overload, severely dropping pH levels even further. The result: an irresistible food source where cell-destroying scavengers such as bacteria, viruses, and parasites love to live and breed.

These scavengers and their potent acidic waste by-products called mycotoxins further compromise pH and create disruptions in the body's bio-systems. This is what the medical community refers to as metabolic or degenerative disease. It is a vicious, cascading cycle in which one acid condition creates another. Low oxygen, an acidic diet, nutrition-

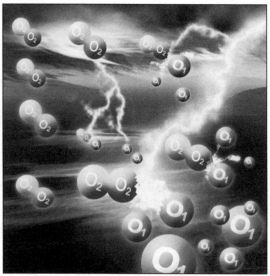

al deficiencies, and toxic emotions create acid pH in the cells, triggering acid-producing mycotoxic waste from bacteria and parasites.

In the book, **Flood Your Body With Oxygen**, Ed McCabe makes the following statement: *"I have been telling everyone for many years that the ultimate cause of ALL disease is a LACK OF ENOUGH OXYGEN to clean our inner fluid environments. This lack of oxygen allows two major causes of all disease to overcome us: Toxic build-ups, and the formation of various colonies of microorganisms inside us, especially in the blood. The toxins poison us, and the organisms eat us while dispersing more toxins."* (2)

As the cells become deprived of necessary nutrients, the entire body begins to rot and decay from the inside out. Bacteria, viruses, fungus, spores, parasites, and other microorganisms breed, while hardened mucous and decomposed waste products continue to accumulate and fester. An overly acidic body starts to eat away at tissue like battery acid eating away at skin tissue, slowly corroding and debilitating the entire body. The body eliminates what it can and the remainder settles in the weakest cells that are not strong enough to clean house.

I say that disease comes from the inside out, not the outside in. It is the state of the body's biological terrain that acts as the catalyst for development and progression of all "dis-ease" – not germs or pathogens. This does not ignore or preclude additional contributing factors from external trauma, airborne microforms, air pollution, radiation, chemicals, and drugs. These also provide negative impressions on the genes within the cell. Unless overridden, "dis-ease" is the response that invariably develops by the signaling of negative gene expressions.

If left unchecked, these acidic wastes will interrupt all life-sustaining cellular activities and functions – anything from the beating of your heart to the neuro-firing of your brain. Over-acidification interferes with life itself, leading to all sickness and the one "dis-ease" – **CELLULAR MALFUNCTION**

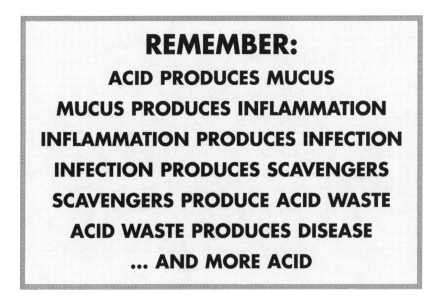

REMEMBER:

ACID PRODUCES MUCUS
MUCUS PRODUCES INFLAMMATION
INFLAMMATION PRODUCES INFECTION
INFECTION PRODUCES SCAVENGERS
SCAVENGERS PRODUCE ACID WASTE
ACID WASTE PRODUCES DISEASE
... AND MORE ACID

Pharmaceutical Drugs Perpetuate
An Acid Condition

During the height of this degrading acid cycle, numerous symptoms will manifest in the body. Sadly, it's at this stage that people run to their doctor for help. There are no pharmaceutical drugs in existence that can reverse this acidic process. In fact, no pharmaceutical drug neutralizes acids or increases pH. Pharmaceuticals only create more acids, worsening the problem and contributing to the acid demise. No pharmaceutical drugs address or correct nutritional deficiencies, especially when it comes to deficiencies of alkaline minerals. They only rob nutrients and antioxidants from the body. There are no pharmaceutical drugs that can boost or modulate the immune system; they only destroy or compromise it.

The fact is pharmaceutical drugs *do not cure* any degenerative, metabolic or autoimmune disease. How could they? By their very nature they are poisonous, acidic, and destructive – not nutritive, alkaline building and constructive. This is particularly true with antibiotics, chemotherapy and HCL derivatives. Why do you think there are multiple side effects associated with all pharmaceuticals? How can you treat an acid condition with another acid, namely pharmaceuticals? This would be like trying to cure someone who accidentally ingests a poison with another poison.

Disease and symptoms are separate entities. Medical science teaches that they are one in the same, and that by removing the symptom you somehow eliminate the disease. Disease is not an object that you go to war against or kill. It is a slow, degenerative acidic process that incubates over time. The fact of the matter is most doctors are <u>drugging the symptoms</u> of a collective cellular cry – individual cells, screaming in unison from excess acidity and nutritional deficiencies. The symptoms are not the problem. Headaches, nausea, fever, skin rashes, brain fog, severe exhaustion, gastric bloating, angina pain, and dizziness are all the body's intelligent warning signals of a compromised cellular engine problem; an organ or system bogged down with excess acids and toxins from circulation, respiration, and elimination problems.

Suppressing symptoms with "anti" medication is analogous to snipping the wire to a blinking oil light on your car's

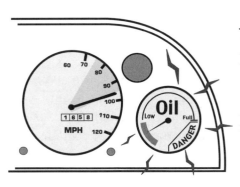

dashboard thinking you just fixed the engine, instead of lifting up the hood and putting oil in your engine so the light goes off. Allopathic or conventional physicians look at the blinking warning light, not the engine, as the problem. They treat the symptoms of your cellular engine malfunction, not the actual bogged down, clogged cellular engine problem stemming from toxicities and insufficiencies.

The big problem with our present medical system is that it is geared toward recognizing disease only when it has reached crisis proportions. This is like saying that a fire is only a fire when the flames have burst through the roof, when, in reality, the real fire started from the cigarette butt that began smoldering in the couch. How would you perceive a fireman spraying the smoke (symptom) billowing out of the windows believing he is putting out the fire?

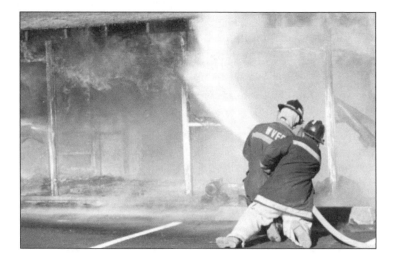

The drug companies tell you straight out that they are going against your body's self-healing mechanisms by the names and contraindications of their drugs. The mainstream philosophy of palliative drug treatments do not cure, nor can they. They are suppressive, counterproductive, and antagonistic in nature, and for this reason they are called "anti" – meaning against (i.e. **anti**biotics, **anti**diuretics, **anti**depressants, **ant**acids, **anti**anxiety agents, **anti**histamines, **anti**-inflammatories, **anti**-hypertensives, etc.). All "anti" medications work against the body's healing systems, not with it, and for this reason have multiple side effects. You cannot suppress, manipulate or mimic one body system without throwing off three or four more systems.

In reality, pharmaceutical drugs are a disease. Side effects are direct effects. For example, if you have a headache and you take codeine or another analgesic and an aggravated side effect of a bleeding ulcer occurs, you have another disease. If you have fluid retention due to dehydration and you take a diuretic drug that vacuums out all your potassium and electrolytes triggering cardiac arrest or fibrillations, the diuretics caused a new disease. If pharmaceutical research were the exact science they claim it to be, why does every drug have multiple side effects?

This absurd, twisted pseudo-science called pharmacology originated from the Germ Theory of Disease perpetrated by Louis Pasteur in the late 1800s. It has continued to this day in all medical school training with little to no opposition. What makes Pasteur's Germ Theory so believable is that it seems to make common sense. Killing bacteria with antibiotics against such strains as staphylococcal, streptococci, bacilli and pneumonia seemed to be the panacea in the 1950s, but all it did was set up shop for stronger enemy-resistant strains to battle in the future.

Bacteria and viruses are the secondary, not primary, causes of disease. In their ignorance, the medical establishment has created their own business by shoving disease deeper into a chronic state with drugs that suppress symptoms. This will eventually require more radical trauma procedures and mutilating surgeries in the future because they never address the acidic state of the patient or the root causes of disease.

Patients become trapped in a medical merry-go-round of more office visits, more prescriptions, more MRIs, more CAT Scans, more chemo, more radiation, and more surgery. This brain-dead mentality of suppressing symptoms in order to treat disease has been going on since the indoctrination (in-doctor-ination) of pharmaceutical medicine almost a century ago. This false religious doctrine, taught by atheistic professors at top medical institutions, needs a paradigm shift in order to bring back true healing sciences.

Often in today's world of medicine and pharmaceutical monopolies, scientific proof falls under the title of who wants it most, how much you can pay, and how fast do you need it. Being a Nutritional Scientist and Independent Researcher myself, it is blatantly clear to me that scientists' findings are based upon false premises, biased research, personal philosophies, and financial loyalty to the drug companies rather than on truly scientific, verifiable data.

Sink Or Swim

Dr. Robert Young, one of the world's foremost experts on the subject of pH and cellular health, authored the book **Sick And Tired? Reclaim Your Inner Terrain.** In it he gives an excellent analogy of how we poison our bodies daily and disrupt the critical acid/alkaline balance necessary for health:

"Think of your body as a fish tank. Think of the importance of maintaining the integrity of the internal fluids of the body that we 'swim' in daily. Imagine the fish in this tank are your cells and organ systems bathed in the fluids, which transport food and remove waste. Now, imagine I back up my car and put the tailpipe up against the air intake filter supplying oxygen to the water in the tank. The water becomes filled with carbon monoxide, lowering the pH, creating an acidic environment, and threatening the health of the fish, your cells and organs. What if I throw in too much food or the wrong kind of food and the fish are unable to consume or digest it all, and it starts to decompose and putrefy? Toxic waste chemicals build up as the food breaks down, creating more acidic by-products, altering the optimum pH. Well, basically, this is a small example of what we are doing to our internal fluids every day, some of us more than others. We are fouling our internal fluids with pollution (smoking?), drugs, excessive intake of food, over-consumption of acid forming foods, and any number of other transgressions which compromise the delicate balance of pH that maintains homeostasis. Some of us have fish tanks (bod-

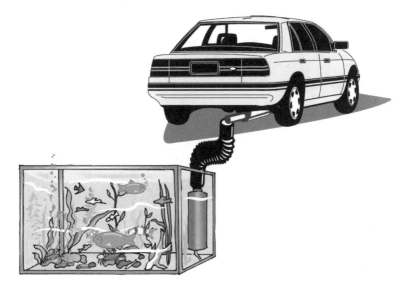

ies) that are barely able to support life, yet we somehow manage to struggle from day to day building more severe imbalances until there is the inevitable crash and debilitating chronic, disturbing, and disorganized symptomatology to deal with." (3)

Violating Common Sense Principles of Health

Most people in today's world still have a hazy idea about what constitutes disease. They believe it to be something mysterious that attacks them from the outside and that there is very little they can do about it. So in their confusion, they run to their doctor for every ache and pain, cold, cough, fever, or rash, expecting some sort of magic "silver bullet" prescription pill to cure every ill before they leave the office.

We're constantly violating almost every fundamental principle of life when it comes to nourishing the body temple and how we should live here on earth. We blindly accept the medical profession's atheistic teachings as to why we get sick and then we accept their drugs, chemotherapy, radiation, and surgery as the only means of treating the sickness. Sadly, their treatments only make us sicker, more acidic, more immuno-suppressed, and more nutritionally deprived, which exhausts our savings and slowly kills us. Why is it that we never question the validity of their teachings?

We violate sound principles of health by what we feed our bodies and minds, and then when they break down, we violate the same principles again as we poison ourselves further by trusting the medical deity in an attempt to get healthy. What in modern medicine's toolbox establishes a healthy alkaline environment to the cells? The answer is nothing! Physicians are limited to cutting out body parts, poisoning the body with prescription drugs, and using toxic chemotherapy and lethal radiation. Re-establishing health to the patient is the **only** way to reverse disease. Health cures disease, not drugs. Research into synthetic, petroleum-based, carbon chain pharmaceutical constructs will never be able to establish health within a patient.

The path of least resistance for the body is a natural state of health that calls for the least amount of energy and electrical force expended. The body fights to maintain healthy balance and homeostasis 24-hours a day. Health is God's path of least resistance. The truth is the laws of health cannot be broken. We can only break ourselves against them.

God's laws of health and vitality are set in motion just like the law of gravity. If you attempt to break the law of gravity by jumping out of a 10-story window, you will only break yourself against a slab of concrete and *illustrate* the law of gravity in action. The same is true for any-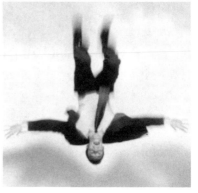

one who goes against the law of pH-based health by continued ingestion of acid-producing foodless foods, toxic beverages, pharmaceuticals, industrial contaminants, and long-term stress. You have to go against the grain of the self-healing systems sometimes for decades to manifest sickness and disease.

The Chemical Make-Up of Our Bodies

If you were to examine a decomposed body buried for decades in the soil, you will find that the remains are truly the soil-based elements that make up "the dust of the ground." We have a book written thousands of years ago telling us that the building materials of man are derived from the elements contained in the earth and atmosphere.

"And the LORD God formed man of the Dust of the Ground, and breathed into his nostrils the breath of life; and man became a living soul." **(Genesis 2:7)**

Science has only recently discovered through spectromography and graphite furnace lab analysis what the Bible has been telling us for thousands of years. It is clear that man is primarily made of the airborne elements of oxygen, carbon, nitrogen and hydrogen (over 96%) – the breath of life – while the remaining 4%, the basic minerals such as potassium, magnesium, calcium, silver, copper and gold, etc, come from the earth – the dust of the ground. These same building materials are necessary for maintaining healthy blood, tissues and cell alkalinity. If we analyze the molecular structure of all proteins, we find a combination of oxygen, carbon, nitrogen and hydrogen. Carbohydrates are carbon/hydrate, meaning carbon plus a water molecule. Fats, triglycerides and vitamins are also carbon, hydrogen nitrogen, and oxygen combinations.

This book is based on the simplicity of reversing all disease processes by balancing pH, which naturally stimulates our own built-in, self-healing, autogenic systems. It is in direct opposition to man's "kill mentality" and weapons of war, which are acidic, temporary, and insidiously destructive to organs and systems.

The average person has ignorantly conformed to this world in almost every area dealing with the physical body. We grab food at fast food restaurants, shop at conventional grocery stores, and "eat out" in restaurants 75% of the time. We are now paying an extremely heavy penalty. Due to our disobedience, ignorance, and laziness, millions of people are afflicted with a record number of health ailments. We would be wise to turn back to the simple prescriptions for health that are outlined for us in the scriptures.

"If thou wilt diligently hearken to the voice of the LORD thy God, and will do that which is right in his sight, and wilt give ear to his commandments, and keep all his statutes, I will put none of the diseases upon thee, which I have brought upon the Egyptians: FOR I AM THE LORD THAT HEALETH THEE." **(Exodus 15:26)**

So, in short, sickness and disease are simply the result of our body's natural reaction to the foreign acids and toxins to which we so frequently expose them.

The Simplicity of Creation

Our Creator is a God of simplicity, not complexity. If anything in this world is built on confusion, chaos and mystery, it is not of the LORD, it is of the evil one. What do you think the medical profession is built on? Confusion, chaos and mystery!!! Their strategy is to get you to believe that there are 10,001 different diseases all needing outside intervention from drugs and surgery, when the truth is that there is only one disease – CELLULAR MALFUNCTION.

As Dr. Robert O. Young so eloquently expressed in his book, **Sick and Tired? Reclaim Your Inner Terrain:** *"There is only one physiological disease – the over-acidification of the body, due primarily to an inverted way of eating and living. This over-acidification leads to the one sickness, or primary symptom – the overgrowth in the body of microorganisms, whose poisons produce the symptoms we call 'diseases'."* (3)

Disease is nothing more than the outworking of the natural law of autogenesis – a natural, self-propelling process of the body's inherent ability to remove toxic accumulation in and around the cells. Its removal methods are the uncomfortable purgings we know as diarrhea, vomiting, sweating, coughing, runny nose and fever that usually keep us running to the doctor. Every symptom is proof of the innate intelligence God has bestowed upon the human body to purge, excrete, or flush poisonous waste through one or more of our elimination channels: via the skin, colon, nose, lungs, ears, and urinary tract.

Pasteur's Germ Theory of Disease was Mistaken Science

Like dogs chasing their own tails, scientists go cross-eyed looking at elephants under a <u>microbe</u>-scope to discover new disease-causing germs – despite the fact that germs and microorganisms do not cause disease all by their microscopic selves. They only take advantage of us when our bodies are in a weakened/compromised state, burdened by toxins. Sickness is not caused by bacteria, but bacteria come with the sickness.

Enlightened understanding demonstrates that germs are not the cause of disease any more than flies, maggots, and rats cause garbage. Flies, maggots and rats do not *cause* garbage, they feed on it. These scavengers, who seek their own habitat, show up as an aftermath *as a result of the garbage.*

That's why I refer to Louis Pasteur's *"Germ Theory of Disease"* as the *"Rat Theory of Garbage."* If germs cause disease, then rats must cause garbage. Show me a building full of rats, and I'll show you a building that's full of garbage with sanitation problems. Show me a person who has accumulated waste matter in organs and tissues, low oxygen levels, weakened immunity, nutritional deficiencies, and an acidic pH environment, and I will show you cancer, bacterial, viral, fungal, and parasitic infections.

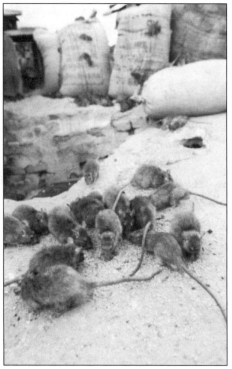

Many well-respected, cellular terrain specialists in the fields of cell physiology, microbiology, disease pathology and molecular biology, have all proven, beyond a shadow of a doubt many decades ago, that germs don't cause disease, they develop in response to the inner condition of the cellular environment. So why would mainstream science continue their research in the wrong direction based upon Pasteur's false Germ Theory of Disease, when it has long been proven that germs and bacteria are secondary, not primary causes of disease?

It's because around it exists a colossal infrastructure of commercial interests that supports a trillion dollar industry, based solely upon this pseudo-science. Until medical science comes to grips with this reality, they will be chasing their tails around in the dark for another hundred years. The entire medical establishment has built their house of cards on Pasteur's false doctrine. It's ironic and indeed pathetic that human beings, the highest form of intelligence on this planet, have managed to build the vast pharmaceutical industry on the central purpose of poisoning and attacking the lowest forms of life on the planet – GERMS!

Dr. M.L. Leverson, M.D., Ph.D., M.A., an American physician practicing during Pasteur and Béchamp's era discovered some of Antoine Béchamp's writings in New York and realized that Pasteur had plagiarized Béchamp. Upon this discovery Leverson went to France and personally met with Béchamp where he heard the story of plagiarism first hand. After that meeting, he has done a great deal to bring Béchamp's work to public attention. Here is what Leverson had to say about Pasteur as it's quoted in the book, **The Dream and Lie of Louis Pasteur**:

"...the entire fabric of the germ theory of disease rests upon assumptions which not only have not been proved, but which are incapable of proof, and many of them can be proved to be the reverse of truth. The basic one of these unproven assumptions, the credit for which in its present form is wholly due to Pasteur, is the hypothesis that all the so called infectious and contagious disorders are caused by germs, each disease having its own specific germ, which germs have existed in the air from the beginning of things, and that though the body is closed to these pathogen's germs when in good health, when the vitality is lowered the body becomes susceptible to their inroads." (4)

Dr. Robert O. Young, in his book, **The pH Miracle**, explained his take on the germ theory as follows:

*"Overacidification of body fluids and tissues underlies **all** disease, and general 'dis-ease' as well. For one thing, it is only when it is acidic that the body is vulnerable to germs – in a healthy base balance, germs can't get a foothold. Furthermore, acids are the expression of all sickness and disease."* (5)

Antoine Béchamp Was
The Real Scientific Genius

The most profound discovery of the late 19th and early 20th century, with the exception of the incredible inventions made by the brilliant Nikola Tesla, was the discovery of tiny living ferments present in all cells and body fluids. Top French scientist, Antoine Béchamp, termed these tiny living ferments *"microzymas."* Later they were called *"protits"* by Günter Enderlein, a renowned German scientist, and *"somatids"* by Dr. Gaston Naessens, an elite French microbiologist. (2)

Antoine Béchamp (1816-1908) had a scientific mind to understand and unravel the disease process unlike any other. His credentials included being a Master of Pharmacy, Doctor of Science, Doctor of Medicine, Professor of Medical Chemistry and Pharmacy, Fellow and Professor of Physics and Toxicology, Professor of Biological Chemistry, and Dean of the Faculty of Medicine. He was a research scientist up until his death at the age of 91. Upon his death, it took eight pages of the national science journal of France just to list the titles of his scientifically published works in 1908. Unfortunately for Béchamp, Louis Pasteur (1822-1895) had deep political pull and incredibly wealthy business associates with global connections. These cronies were not interested in health care, but management of sickness at the expense of human lives. They were interested in establishing a new global enterprise to control medicine and disease like some kind of commodity, in hopes of profiting trillions of dollars from human suffering.

The cover-up of Antoine Béchamp's discoveries has meant untold misery and suffering for the human race by allowing surgical, pharmaceutical, chemotherapy/radiation, and vaccine research development to dominate mainstream medicine. Even Pasteur himself cried out on his deathbed that Claude Bernard, a leading cellular physiologist, was right on target. That is, the germs are nothing, and the cellular terrain is everything.

It's a travesty that Pasteur, who knew that Antoine Béchamp was right, never gave credit where credit was due *(Béchamp's discoveries of pleomorphism and microzymas)*. It was not Pasteur's Germ Theory of monomorphism that should have become the established curriculum in all medical institutions. This distinguished honor and the health of our modern society should have rested on Béchamp's microzymas and pleomorphic principles, that germs change forms based on cellular terrain.

Béchamp Discovered that Germs are A Result of Diseased Tissue, Not Outside Invasion

Antoine Béchamp was able to show scientifically that it isn't the bacteria or the viruses themselves that produce disease; they are an <u>aftermath</u> of diseased tissue. Germs are the chemical by-products of pleomorphic microorganisms acting on the unbalanced, malfunctioning cells and dead tissue that actually produce disease. Disease-associated microorganisms do not produce the disease condition themselves, any more than mosquitoes cause a stagnant swamp. The disease is born out of the acidic, low-oxygen cellular environment, created by a toxic diet, toxic environmental exposures, toxic emotions, and a toxic lifestyle. This sup-

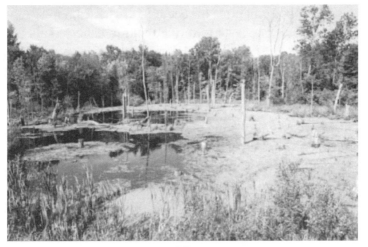

ports the morbid changes of germs to bacteria, bacteria to viruses, viruses to fungal forms and fungal forms to cancer cells. Had Béchamp's breakthrough discoveries been incorporated into current medical curriculum, we would have already been experiencing the virtual elimination of disease and the end of the pharmaceutical industry.

Microzymas: The Intelligent Life Force of Nature

The foundation of all life on earth revolves around tiny indestructible living entities that Antoine Béchamp called microzymas. "Micro" meaning small or tiny and "zymas" referring to a special class of immortal enzymes. According to Béchamp, microzymas exist in every cell and all bodily fluids and they have an innate intelligence that communicates genetic information to the cell to produce either life-giving pathogens (LIVE) or death-giving pathogens (EVIL/VILE) depending on the cellular terrain (pH).

It's interesting to note that extreme heat, antibiotics, radiation or any other destructive medical weapon of war cannot destroy these living entities. Since you cannot kill microzymas, bacteria or viruses as I just stated, antibiotics will only trigger resistant strains of these morbid evolutions into stronger forms, such as the transformations of bacteria to viruses, viruses to fungus, fungus to yeast, yeast to mold, mold to cancer. This is what Antoine Béchamp meant when he said that germs were pleomorphic ("Pleo" meaning many, "morph" meaning form – change to many forms).

Microzymas change the face of pathogens like a chameleon. Unfortunately, symptom manipulation with pharmacology and antibiotics creates a magical "shell game" of switching diseases. This creates more serious symptoms and chronic disease conditions, which are totally different from the original disease. They add disease-to-disease, creating job security for the medical money-go-round. This quick-fix drug game of voodoo medicine is what's now causing the disease epidemic in this country. And it is what is making hospitals and doctors the number three killer in the U.S., maiming and killing roughly 400,000 patients per year.

In a state of vibrant health, microzymas harmoniously perform evolved aerobic fermentation, as seen when grapes ferment into wine, or when beneficial gut flora like acidophilus and bifidus, proliferate through fermentation in the gut wall. On the flip side, in a diseased condition, characterized by low oxygen, malnutrition, acid pH, poor circulation, stress, and built up toxins in and around the cells, microzymas signal the cells, alerting them to bring the organism back to the soil (dust of the ground) because the organism itself is debilitated to the point of being sick and dying.

Microscopic germs evolve into yeast, molds, viruses, fungi and other morbid microforms that eat away at the necrotic acid tissue, acting as a clean-up crew. It's the eternal microzymas that are responsible for a dead animal or a leaf from a tree decomposing back to the ground, transferring a cycle of life back to the dust of the earth for future plant growth.

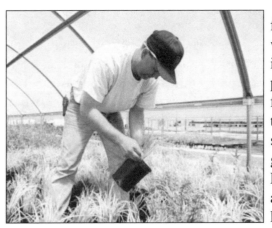 Any organic farmer or gardener will tell you the importance of specific pH conditions for food enzyme fermentation. Without proper soil pH, seeds will not germinate properly. Plants become sick and produce a very low yield. A carbohy-

drate grain like corn has a different pH requirement to make silage, compared with silage made from young grass, which is protein. Farmers often add enzymes and specific bacteria to regulate the pH of different food sources that require fermentation. Similarly, our body's innate intelligence regulates digestive enzymes and bacteria to control the pH of different digestive juices for different foods through electrical impulses from the tongue receptors in the chewing process relayed to the pancreas.

The answer to how disease develops lies in the condition of your cellular terrain, not in outside microbial invasions. An analogy of this is four people in a closed elevator with one sneezing and coughing from a recent cold. Within 24-hours, one of the three on the elevator contracts a head cold, while the other two remain well. What prevented the other two from getting sick? If germs cause sickness, the equal exposure to the rhinovirus from the sneeze would have caused all three to get sick. Disease causing germs need appropriate soil in which to grow. It's all based upon your inner terrain at the time of 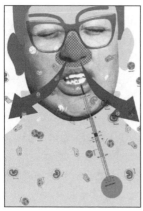 exposure. Is your pH in balance? Will it support the development of unwanted guests, or necessary life-giving pathogens?

In the early stages of acidosis the warning symptoms are mild. They can include lethargy, skin eruptions, headaches, allergies, colds, flu and sinus problems. These symptoms are frequently treated, more accurately "manipulated," with antibiotic drugs and suppressive medications. With continued suppression of an acidic, toxic environment warning signals will lead to more serious symptoms.

The disease is driven deeper into a chronic state through a seven stage process of: **Enervation, Intoxication, Irritation,**

Inflammation, Induration, Ulceration and **Fungation**, which leads to mutation (cancer), where weakened organs and systems start to give out and go into failure, whether it's heart failure, lung failure, thyroid failure, or adrenal burn-out.

My view is that the toxins, basically acids from the microforms, combine to provoke the body into producing symptoms of a healing crisis. The body tends to purge or eliminate the toxic residues: from the nose through a runny nose, the skin through sweat, the colon through diarrhea, increased respiration of CO_2 through the lungs. Remember – it's not the pathogens themselves that initiate disease – they only show up as an aftermath of an acidic, compromised, cellular terrain.

Inevitably the immune system is compromised as a result. Then medical doctors come in and treat the acid condition with other acids (antibiotics/pharmaceuticals) to knock out the warning symptoms of your acute, cellular cry: "I'm acidic," your body is saying.

The Seven Stages of Disease Progression

In order to better understand the entire progression of disease, I want to expound on the seven-stage process that I just mentioned, beginning with mild symptoms and ending in a full-blown crisis. These seven stages are really just symptoms of intelligent body-instituted healing.

1. ENERVATION (ENERVATE): To deprive of nerve, energy, vital force or strength; physical, mental, or moral weakness. Devitalize, and/or weaken.

The first stage of disease progression is Enervation, which can be caused by overeating, drinking too much alcohol, worry, overindulgence of devitalized, refined, processed foods and lifeless, carbonated beverages, excessive sugar intake, salt, coffee, tap water, drugs, polluted air, lack of sleep, stress, and stimulants. The result: cellular congestion, overall weakness, depression, and reduced vital energy or strength.

2. INTOXICATION: The state of being poisoned by a drug or other substance.

The second stage of degeneration is intoxication resulting from the abusive acts of stage one. Over time this slows the body's ability to eliminate poisons, by clogging the detoxification organs and filtration systems of the intestines, liver, kidneys, skin, blood circulation and lymphatic flow.

Our vital energy is always divided between digestion, assimilation, stimulation, cell absorption, and elimination. As more energy is diverted to digest the poisons listed in stage one, while artificial stimulants such as coffee, alcohol, herbal stimulants, sugar, tobacco, inorganic substances, and toxic caffeine are taken in to try and compensate for the loss of energy, cellular energy capacity drastically declines through adrenal exhaustion. This leaves the body intoxicated, sluggish, burned out, and weakened. Continued enervation and intoxication lead to a susceptible crisis named "dis-ease" or what I call the **Medical Twilight Zone** (see chart on page 44). In this zone of "dis-ease" the person is neither healthy nor chronically sick. They are somewhere in between. They have

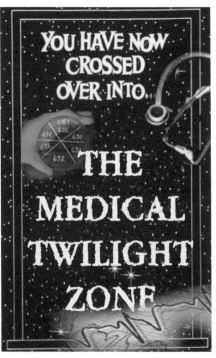

- 40 -

fallen through the cracks of the medical machine with established parameters calibrated specifically for trauma and crisis. Consequently, they are given a clean bill of health.

3. IRRITATION: The bringing of a bodily part or organ to an abnormally excited or sensitive condition.

The third stage of disease progression is due to an excess of acid-forming foods and beverages – from sugars, fried foods, coffee, carbonated beverages, alcohol, red meat, antibiotics, etc. – which results in the body's fluid conditions developing an acid pH. This condition depletes alkaline reserves and over time irritates tissue lining due to the acid wastes. Irritation symptoms can manifest as itching, skin rashes, burning eyes, irritable bowel syndrome, etc. which all cause redness leading to inflammation.

4. INFLAMMATION: The response of your body's tissues to irritation or injury. Inflammation may be acute or chronic. Its chief signs are redness, heat, swelling, and pain, accompanied by loss of function.

The fourth stage of disease progression triggers the onset of inflammation, indicative of accumulated pustulence or dried blood and thick mucous in and around the organs, joints, and cells. This triggers an immune response, causing the white blood cells to spill histamines, cytokines and other inflammatory substances in the fight to clean up the toxemic condition. Continued inflammation through pro-inflammatory hormone release will eventually lead to stone-like formations of trapped inorganic wastes creating a protective barrier in the joints, kidneys, and gall bladder. At this point the body's weakened, enervated filtration organs are unable to expel the accumulated, hardened waste material. Allergies, inflammation, and immuno-suppression are the result.

A so-called allergy is nothing more than the irritation of an already chronically inflamed nasal passage or lung tissue from a pronounced toxemic condition. Toxemia irritation is the basic cause of all inflammation, including in the intestinal lining and the epithelial lining in the lungs. This stage of inflammation is characterized by all the "itises" i.e.: sinusitis, nephritis, hepatitis, meningitis, appendicitis, etc.

5. INDURATION: Hardening of a tissue, particularly the skin, due to excess fluid retention, inflammation, or growth of a tumor to protect the body from further damage.

The fifth stage of degeneration is earmarked by a gradual thickening or hardening of the mucous and sub-mucosal tissues, due to continued inflammation un-resolved by detoxification methods. The increased hardening from solidifying hydrogenated and saturated fats, LDL cholesterol, chlorine, calcium, iron, and other inorganic minerals, chokes arterial circulation, cutting off oxygen and inhibiting nutrient flow to the cells. This hypoxia gives rise to cell apoptosis or programmed cell death. Symptoms of induration include hardening of the arteries, skin eruptions, open sores, ulcers, pustulence, cataracts, cysts, polyps, liver spots, kidney stones, callused feet, calcium spurs and gall stones.

6. ULCERATION: A craterlike skin or mucous membrane lesion; a sore open either to the surface of the body or to a natural cavity, and accompanied by the disintegration of tissue, the formation of pus, etc.

The sixth stage of disease progression is an active degeneration from cell apoplexy – essentially a paralysis of circulatory functions in blood and lymph due to tissue and arterial hardening. Ulceration can manifest as a stress ulcer, a stasis ulcer, a trophic ulcer, a peptic ulcer, even ulcerative colitis. Instead of normal toxin elimination, dried blood and toxic pus erupt from open wounds, boils, fistulas, internal ulcers, or are discharged from the eyes, ears, nose, vagina or other body cavities. Examples of these are cankers associated with AIDS and herpes simplex. Another symptom of ulceration is adrenal exhaustion/stress from a highly toxic, enervated condition.

7. FUNGATION: Excessive overgrowth of fungus in the blood and tissues.

The last and final stage of degeneration is fungation. This condition is an overgrowth of fungus in the body, consisting of molds, mildew, spores, yeasts (candidiasis), and cancer. There are more than a thousand toxins produced by yeast, fungus, and mold, and their acidic wastes contribute directly or indirectly to a wide range of symptoms. In this final stage, there is a cellular disorder from repeated free radical hits on the genetic material, damaging DNA during replication, transcription, and translation of the new cells. This inevitably leads to cell proliferation and mutation of tissue growth to a morbid state. During this final stage, healthy cells no longer renew themselves, but form cancerous mutations. Doing a live blood analysis using darkfield microscopy will easily detect yeast, fungus, mold and cancer cells. This is the stage where microzymas start signaling death to the organism.

All seven progressive stages of disease are nothing more than the body's effort to return to balance and order (homeostatsis), by attempting to purge itself of the unwanted toxins that are poisoning it. The symptoms of this triggered healing crisis are what medical science calls disease.

Acidic pH is the Primary Factor Triggering the Seven Stage Progression of Disease

Too much acidity in the body's tissues and cells is a significant factor in triggering the seven-stage progression of disease. When acid wastes build up within weakened cells and

"Medical Twilight Zone"
Homotoxicology

Dis - Ease — Humoral Phases — Chronic Cellular Phases

	PHASE 1	PHASE 2 Excretion	PHASE 3 Excretion	PHASE 4	PHASE 5	PHASE 6	PHASE 7	PHASE 8	PHASE 9
Category	**Enervation** Physical, Mental + Moral Weakness	**Intoxication** Cellular Toxemia Needing Stimulants	**Irritation** (acidosis) Excitatory Or Sensitive Condition	**Inflammation** Redness, heat, swelling, pain, Dermatitis, Sinusitis	**Induration** Thickening, Hardening, Calcification, Chokes Circulation	**Degeneration** Ulceration Degeneration Of Tissues & Organs	**Fungation** Systemic overgrowth of Fungi	**Trauma**	**Mutation**
Symptoms	Mild Depression, Lethargy, Reduced strength	Sluggish, Depression, Brain fog, Sweating	Nervousness, Irritable Bowel Syndrome, Fever, Coughing, Asthma, Osteoporosis, Peridental Disease	Colitis, Nephritis, Loss of function, Bronchitis, All Itis's	Kidney Stones, Open sores, Ulcers, Pustulence, Calcium spurs, Skin Eruptions	Stress ulcer, Stasis ulcer, Peptic ulcer, Trophic ulcer	Candidiasis, Mold, Cancer Origin, Morbidity	Crisis PET Scan, MRI Scan, Blood Profiles, Cancer Markers, Western Medicine, Calibration Of Diagnostics	DEATH

Perfect Health & Vitality — Atomic & Molecular Disturbance — NO SYMPTOMS

Impregnation Phase

Dedifferentiation neoplasm

SYMPTOMS →

Self Healing Vicariation →

7 Phases of Dis-Ease Progression

organs that are too weak to clean house, a fertile environment exists for disease causing pathogens to breed. When we are born, we have the highest alkaline mineral concentration that gives us perfectly balanced pH. That's why most degenerative, metabolic, and autoimmune diseases do not show up until after 40 or so years of abuse from acidic assaults to the blood, tissues, and cells.

The major underlying factor in all "disease labels" is the accumulation of acid residues in tissues and cells. The accompanying poor blood and lymph circulation, poor cell activity, poor oxygenation, nutritional deficiencies, and dehydration, causes an electrical disturbance at the cellular level. This disorder is what science calls disease; the descriptive name of the particular disease just depends upon the location of the deposited toxins.

So, in short, acute or recurrent infections are either an attempt by the body to mobilize mineral reserves from all parts of the body or crisis attempts to detoxify and eliminate acids. Mucus forms in the colon, lungs and nasal passages to expel them from the body. For example, the lungs will cast out acids by trapping them in mucus, forcing a loose cough to expel them. The skin throws off acids producing symptoms such as eczema, dermatitis, acne, or other skin disorders. Chronic trauma results when all possibilities for neutralizing these toxins have been exhausted.

The Intelligence of Cell Health

Shortly after our father's sperm merges with our mother's fertilized egg at conception, the combined genetic blueprints fuse to create the biological map that coordinates the millions of life-sustaining functions. Trillions of cells simultaneously performing their many tasks in a finely orchestrated dance of life is a miracle beyond our understanding of organization power.

The genetic script that runs the liver's molecular machinery to store and release sugar molecules, synthesize cholesterol, detoxify the blood, secrete bile and digest hemoglobin pigment work in tandem with the colon cells that are simultaneously fermenting aerobic bacteria, absorbing fluid, and propelling yesterday's breakfast along the intestinal tract. All this activity is coordinated by a unified biological intelligence. If it weren't for this divine intelligence contained within every cell, we would be a bag of molecules that would drop to the floor.

The body contains the same biochemicals right before and after death, but the intelligence of life directed by God is what turns our molecular motors into a living, breathing biological machine. Individually each of your molecules is a delicate instrument, but unified they animate a flurry of electro-chemical impulses organized by ranks of molecular switches. These turn on and off at certain intervals when necessary. A healthy body depends upon a high level of negative electromagnetic charge on tissue cells' surfaces. Acidity is actually a positive charge that dampens out these electrical fields, affecting cellular communication.

Unless a treatment actually removes acid toxins from the body and increases oxygen, water, and nutrients, the cure, at best, will only be temporary. Otherwise, the disease is driven deeper into a chronic state. Remember, there's not one drug on the market that reduces the acidity of the body or addresses any kind of nutritional deficiency. The only way to properly treat disease conditions is to alkalize the pH which will dispose acids from your cells, tissues, and organs. There is nothing in mainstream medicine that addresses de-acidification, detoxification, fixing nutritional deficiencies, modulating and boosting the immune system, and increasing full body circulation. For this reason, medical science is a complete failure when it comes to curing any degenerative, metabolic, or autoimmune disease. Without removing toxins and acids from all organs, cells and tissues, the body will not be able to heal completely.

There's a wealth of information about unraveling the disease process in Bruce Fife, N.D's popular book, **The Detox Book**. Here's how Fife explains toxins effect on the cells:

"Given the chance, the body will eliminate harmful toxins that weaken our immune system and cause degenerative conditions to develop. The body will heal, replacing damaged, diseased tissues with new healthy cells. But as long as irritating contaminants [acids] remain in the tissues and new toxins are continually added, recovery is impossible. Surgically removing a cancerous growth, for example, from one part of the body may relieve pain, but will not eliminate the cause of the cancer. The disease-causing factors remain, irritating other tissues, and eventually the cancer returns. Removing the symptoms of disease does not cure the disease. The only way to remove the cause of degenerative disease is to allow the body to cleanse itself. Surgery won't do this, drugs won't do this, radiation won't do this. It has to be done internally." (6)

Our performance of everyday tasks from touching and seeing to breathing and thinking can all be traced to the concerted actions of invisible molecular messengers run by the microzymas.

So what is the engine that drives the microzymas? The answer is pH. If the pH is alkaline, it will direct the microzymas to construct healthy molecules for a healthy immune system, thick strands of hair, tough fingernails, even building strong ligaments and blood vessels. On the flip side, if the pH is acidic, it will direct the microzymas to construct molecules that create weakened fingernails, unhealthy dermis layers, weakened immune cells, frail blood vessels, etc.

Cancer Cell Growth Linked To pH Imbalance

Cancer is a systemic, whole body disease that shows up as a tumor site. It can manifest as a fibrinogen protein wrap, an encapsulation, or a bubble or cocoon of mutated, foreign cells, cysts, pulps, lipomas or fibroids in the body's weakest links or target zones. These zones are the storage bins for excess acids and toxins built up in the blood, a natural protection mechanism preventing metastasizing foreign matter or cancer cells from spilling back into the bloodstream or lymphatic system and spreading secondary tumor sites.

Excess acid wastes that can't be expelled fast enough lead to oxygen deprivation and cell fermentation, where healthy cells begin to rot. These rotting cells and their acids stick together like glue, bonding to healthy neighboring cells, creating a domino effect of fermentation. This acid fermentation process is what we label as cancer. It's my conclusion, based on years of research and study, that cancer is nothing more than an electrical disturbance at the sub-atomic and DNA level caused by oxygen deprivation, dehydration, cellular intoxication, lack of circulation and electrical flow that leads to cell asphyxiation, finally resulting in cell mutation.

This process triggers cellular microzymas to evolve into disease-triggering pathogens that change bacteria to yeast, fungus to candida and molds, and molds to cancer, which then produce acidic mycotoxic waste matter. As Dr. Young says in his book **Sick And Tired: Reclaim Your Inner Terrain**: *"Cancer therefore is a four-letter word -ACID."* (3) This is especially true with lactic acid, a common acid waste product caused by low oxygen levels and yeast and fungus fermentation.

In a speech given at the 1966 Nobel-Laureates Conference in Lindau, Germany, Dr. Otto Warburg stated: *"But, even for cancer, there is only one main cause. Summarized in a few words, the prime cause of cancer is the replacement of the respiration of oxygen in normal body cells by a fermentation of sugar."*

The growth of cancer cells is initiated by a fermentation process, which can only be triggered in the absence of oxygen at the cellular level. Just as overworked muscle cells manufacture lactic acid by-products as waste, cancer cells spill lactic acid and other acidic compounds that greatly impact your pH balance. At the same conference Warburg also made the following statements:

"To prevent cancer it is therefore proposed first to keep the speed of the bloodstream so high that the venous blood still contains sufficient oxygen; second, to keep high the concentration of hemoglobin in the blood;..."

"All normal cells meet their energy needs by the respiration of oxygen, whereas cancer cells meet their energy needs in great part by fermentation. From the standpoint of chemistry and physics of life this difference between normal and cancer cells is so great that one can scarcely picture a greater difference. Oxygen gas, the donor of energy in plants and animals is dethroned in the cancer cells and replaced by an energy yielding reaction of the lowest forms, namely a fermentation of glucose."

When you hold your breath, you shut off your oxygen supply and carbon monoxide builds up as an acid waste. If you hold it long enough, you'll eventually die from asphyxiation. When your body's oxygen supply cuts off, your body's blood pH can dip below seven and you will go into a coma or death will result.

The blood performs a balancing act in order to maintain the blood pH within a safe range of 7.30 - 7.45. Some cells, instead of dying as normal cells do in an acid environment, may adapt and survive by becoming abnormal, sugar-metabolizing primitive cells, like yeast. These malignant renegade cells do not communicate with brain function, or with our own DNA memory code. Therefore, malignant cells grow indefinitely and without order to disorder and chaos. This biological disorder is what science calls cancer. So unless an oncologist focuses on de-acidification, detoxification, oxygenation, immune system modulation, hormone regulation, and nutritional assimilation, his or her treatment modalities will be as futile as sweeping back the ocean with a broom.

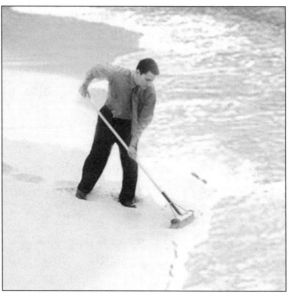

In his book **Healing Celebrations**, Dr. Leonard Horowitz simplified the complexities of cancer by also linking it to acid pH: *"Finally, body acidity, poor circulation, and low oxygen levels go hand in hand. These co-factors all contribute to cancer as well as many other diseases. Cancers, for instance, typically grow in areas with poor circulation. Men get prostate cancers, and women get breast cancers in glands where blood flow is commonly restricted, oxygen levels fall, and acids build up. Colon cancers are linked likewise to over acidity wherein undigested foods ferment. This progressively creates more and more toxicity and acidity in the gut."* (7)

Diabetes and Acid

The pancreas produces one of the highest pH body fluids, pancreatic juice, with a pH of 8.8. A shortage of calcium ions in the body impairs the production and release of the hormone insulin. This can eventually lead to an acidic blood condition. Accumulated acidic waste coats the receptor sites of the insulin producing beta cells, preventing insulin from being synthesized or utilized. The end result is labeled diabetes. An alkaline diet, a detoxification program, and the introduction of nutrients that support insulin production inside the beta cell factories can improve diabetes.

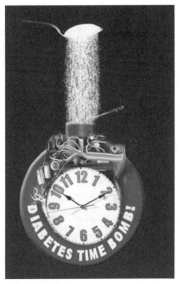

Acidity a Major Culprit in Kidney Disease

As acidic waste products accumulate in the blood, the kidneys, the bloodstream's filter can become taxed and inefficient, leading to kidney stones, nephritis, uremic poisoning and bladder diseases. Most kidney problems can be improved by whole body detoxification and an alkaline diet. In Felicia Drury Kliment's book, **The Acid-Alkaline Balance Diet**, the cause of kidney stones and ultimately most kidney diseases is eloquently explained:

"Kidney stones are usually composed of calcium and oxalic acid. (Urates from uric acid and sulphates from sulphuric acid have also been found in stones.) What most people with kidney stones don't know is that oxalic acid, like calcium, is vital to metabolic function. Ninety-eight percent of the oxalic acid in the body is produced internally and is used for moving food through

the digestive tract by peristalsis (the contraction and expansion of muscles). Oxalic acid also aids in the absorption of calcium into the cells.

"Leftover oxalic acid, along with excess calcium, is removed from the blood by the kidneys, and passes into the urine. Calcium oxalate permeates the urine generally, <u>but only in those people whose urine is overloaded with acidic waste does it form stones.</u>

"It would seem therefore that the way to prevent kidney stones would be to alkalize the urine. But urologists, unaware apparently that the acid-alkaline pH factor in the urine determines whether or not the stones are formed, recommend reducing the levels of calcium and oxalic acid in the diet. Kidney stone patients are instructed not to eat any green vegetables, especially broccoli, which is high in calcium, and spinach, beet greens, and chard because of their high oxalic acid content. By doing so, doctors are depriving their patients of valuable nutrients, one of which, calcium, actually helps prevent kidney stones by alkalinizing the urine." (8)

Acidity Plays a Role in Allergy Problems

Millions of people suffer from allergies caused by every day exposures to agents such as dust mites, cat dander, and pollens. Many foods also play a role in allergies. All of these allergenic agents can cause asthma, nasal and sinus allergies, hives, and even severe, life-threatening anaphylactic reactions. Allergens also prevalent in the workplace include PCB's, turpentine, asbestos, natural rubber latex, benzene, polyurethane, petroleum, and other reactive chemicals. Asthma is one of the more serious problems that can be caused by work-related allergy. It can create recurrent attacks of wheezing, chest tightness, shortness of breath, and coughing symptoms, which can be severe and even disabling. While many of these problems cannot be linked exclusively to acidic pH, evidence suggests allergies and asthma can often be prevented or minimized when pH balancing is incorporated.

Allergies are actually symptoms of an irritation/inflammation reaction due to histamine release, cytokines, prostaglandins, and other inflammatory chemicals that occur as a "healing crisis." Most allergies occur when the body's toxic threshold has been breached. A good analogy here is a tripped fuse in your home. Suppose you turn on every light and appliance in your home and leave them on all day. Later, you flip a switch in your office to turn on your computer and the power goes out in the whole house. Was it the tiny computer switch that caused the blackout, or the total overload of electricity that caused the failure? With allergies, it's that one extra little stress that becomes the straw that breaks the camel's back, once the immune and detox systems reach their total toxic threshold.

I usually find that when you detoxify the body through a powerful cleansing program and ingest beneficial cleansing substances such as wheat grass or fresh vegetable juice, then sinus swelling, runny nose, skin reactions, tearing eyes, and other detox reactions of eliminating acid toxins eventually disappear. Yeast and fungus, whose poisons are acid, may contribute significantly to your hay fever and sneezing. If you have no symptomatic yeast or fungus, it would be virtually impossible for you to manifest allergies. Remember, it's the toxic acidic inner terrain coupled with a weakened immune system that triggers allergic response.

Obesity Is Linked To Acid pH

If tissue pH deviates too far to the acid side, a lack of oxygen will occur, with decelerating cellular metabolism leading to obesity. Acidity, toxicity, dehydration, malnutrition, circulation problems, and lack of oxygen are the ideal cellular environmental condition for lowered metabolic rate.

Over-ingestion of carbohydrates and fats, without enough exercise to burn them as fuel, causes the body to store them as fatty acids. A combination of a sedentary lifestyle (which reduces oxygen), toxic acidic residues and infiltration of morbid microforms in and around the cells, along with the resulting reduction in energy burning ATP, leads to obesity through a lowered metabolic rate.

What is the makeup of this stored, excess weight? The answer is fatty acids. Acetic acid, lactic acid and LDL cholesterol, the derivatives of fatty acid, lower the pH of body fluids drastically. This prevents the cellular engines from burning on all cylinders, reducing metabolic rate. With a reducing metabolic rate, the body does not dispose of unburned food, which is then stored until it can be burned at a later time. To a point, fat is a reservoir of future energy, waiting to be burned. However, if later never comes, we keep adding to the fatty acid reservoir.

Acid coagulates blood capillary beds so there is not much blood flow around fat. These fatty acids generally form under the skin as the dreaded cellulite, piling up on men's waistline and packing onto women's hips, thighs and breasts. Compare the face of an old woman with that of a young woman, and you can see the result of the gradual build up of fat, lower blood flow and reduced skin elasticity. When you truly understand the process of aging and obesity, you will have the incentive to drink alkaline beverages and eat alkaline foods that burn quickly. Anything you can do to help your body dispose of acidic waste on a regular basis should be a priority.

Heart Disease and Stroke Related to Excess Acid

Heart disease and stroke are, respectively, the first and fourth leading causes of death in the United States. Probably no surprise, acids are the principal causes of cardiovascular disease and premature death, as well as major causes of disability.

According to statistics published by the Centers for Disease Control and Prevention (CDC):

"In 2001, 700,142 people died of heart disease (52% of them women), accounting for 29% of all U.S. deaths. The age–adjusted death rate was 246 per 100,000 population. Heart disease is the leading cause of death for American Indians and Alaska Natives, blacks, Hispanics, and whites. Although cancer is the leading cause of death for Asians and Pacific Islanders (accounting for 26.4% of all deaths), heart disease is a close second (25.4%). Heart disease death rates per 100,000 population for the five largest U.S. racial/ethnic groups are as follows: Hispanics, 73; Asians and Pacific Islanders, 77; American Indians, 79; blacks, 210; and whites, 263. In 2004, heart disease is projected to cost $238.6 billion, including health care services, medications, and lost productivity." (9)

So what's causing this epidemic of heart disease and stroke that's killing so many every year? Recent evidence suggests that certain viruses such as the cytomegalovirus, Chlamydia, Herpes simplex virus combined with various forms of virulent bacteria may play a major role in the build-up of plague in arteries. If we were to give credence to Pasteur's "Germ Theory", then killing the bacteria or the virus in the bloodstream would seem to be the cure. Without looking at the acidic condition of the patient, however, medical science will never get to the root cause of this problem. As I have already explained many times throughout this book, when the body's cells and tissues become acidic, this sets up a breeding ground for anaerobic pathogens, which invade the whole body, including the blood vessels. This pathogenic mess spills into the blood and wreaks havoc on the body's cardiovascular system.

In **The Acid Alkaline Balance Diet,** Kliment explained this link as follows: *"Several studies support the connection between the presence of the virus (cytomegalovirus) and the regrowth of plaque. In one study of 75 patients who had had an angioplasty, fatty plaque recurred in 75% of those patients who* *were infected with the cytomegalovirus, while only 8% who were not infected had a recurrence of plaque."* (10)

It's my belief that plaque is a built-in protection system that keeps the viruses, bacteria and acids from killing you on the spot. Without plaque build up, these acids and pathogens would bore right through blood vessels and arterial walls, causing stroke or hemorrhage.

Kliment also goes on to explain the acidic link to cardio-vascular disease:

"Acidic waste in the blood makes scratches and tears on the inside walls of the blood vessels. The injured cells die off and turn into acidic waste, adding to the accumulation of acidic waste in the blood from undigested food debris. The larger the quantities of acidic waste the more rapidly germs multiply, forcing the immune system to defend the walls of the arteries and veins by triggering the growth of tumors to encapsulate germ colonies, patching injuries in the lining of the vessels with fatty plaques to prevent life-threatening leaks, and reacting to arterial degeneration the same way it does to bodily injury from accidents – by triggering the flow of blood to the area which inflames the walls of the arteries. These measures prevent imminent death, but set up the conditions for a heart attack. All that has to occur is for a blood clot to form, which blocks the flow of blood to the heart." (10)

If the overload is too great for the blood, excess acid is dumped into the tissues and cells for storage. Then the lymphatic system and immune system must neutralize what they can and attempt to discharge the toxic waste through one of the elimination routes. If the lymphatic system is overloaded, generally due to a lack of exercise and circulatory problems, acid deposits will suffocate the cells and damage DNA. If the lymphatic system is pumping normally through exercise or massage, it will pick up the acid wastes and neutralize them through the kidneys and liver. Unfortunately, though, in the body it's GI, GO – garbage in, garbage out. These wastes get dumped right back into the blood-stream where they wait in line before elimination, causing a Herxheimer reaction (detoxification symptoms). This will force the blood to try to gather more alkaline salts in order to compensate, often stressing the liver and kidneys.

Although there are other factors involved with cardiovascular disease, certainly the acidic link cannot be overlooked. Running a simple pH test and having your blood checked using darkfield microscopy will tell you in seconds what's going on in your body and whether or not you're vulnerable for a heart attack or stroke. It's important to follow through on all the protocols I've outlined throughout this book for prevention of cardiovascular disease – before it's too late and you're hindered from reaching your full life expectancy.

Gastro-Intestinal Disorders Linked To Excess Acidity

Most stomach disorders – indigestion, nausea, bloating, gastric reflux, etc. – are symptoms caused by pH imbalance and excess acidity in the gastric region. The neutralizing of acid through ingestion of alkaline water, pancreatic acids, plant-based enzymes, alkaline green foods, and alkaline minerals will help to alleviate the acid-related intestinal disorders, including ulcers, without taking destructive Band-Aid agents like antacids and Ibuprofen.

Most Forms of Arthritis Can Be Relieved By Changing pH

The term arthritis simply means "inflammation of the joint" and is used to describe more than 100 rheumatic diseases that cause pain, stiffness, and swelling. Many cases of arthritis are caused by accumulated acid deposits in the joints and wrists. It is this accumulated acid that damages cartilage and coats the cells that produce the lubricating synovial fluids and bursa fluids, causing a dryness which irritates and swells the joints. In the book, **Body Balance, Vitalize Your Health with pH Power,** author Karta Purkh Khalsa, C.D.-N., R.H provides hope to the roughly 43 million Americans afflicted with arthritis:

"Previously, Osteoarthritis (OA) was thought to be a progressive, degenerative disorder and was widely known as 'wear-and-tear arthritis.' It was presumed that everyone, if they lived long enough, would fall prey to OA. It is now known, however, that the disease can be arrested or reversed. Recent evidence has changed the thinking about the disease progress of OA. We now know that the joint cartilage of patients with OA is highly metabolically active. The damaged cartilage tissue actually tries to remodel and repair itself. Though once thought to be impossible, arresting or reversing the disease occurs spontaneously in some OA patients." (11)

In my years of research I've discovered that detoxification protocols, coupled with an alkalizing diet and beneficial supplements such as glucosamine, chondroitin, ginger root, Boswellia, and MSM, will usually relieve arthritis within a very short period of time.

Gout is Linked to Excess Acidity

Gout is an arthritic disease resulting from an excess of uric acid crystals in the blood. It results from inadequate digestion of red meat, seafood, alcohol and poultry. The uric acid salts tend to deposit in the surrounding tissues of the feet, hands and toes. This causes swelling and severe pain, especially in the big toe, due to the broken-glass-like structure of the uric acid crystals. The only solution for gout in mainstream medicine is deadly painkillers and anti-inflammatories, which are both acidic and even more irritating to the joints. Unfortunately, the joints have limited blood circulation to carry out the acid wastes. Un-concentrated cherry juice, an alkaline diet, and increased circulation will help relieve gout symptoms by removing the uric acid crystals.

Excess Acid Can Effect The Eyes

We generally do not attribute changes in our vision to acid conditions. As we accumulate phosphates and urates in our cells, the cells lose more oxygen. This causes unburned sugar in the cell to bond to protein molecules, with the end result being cells and tissues that are stiff, hard and inflexible. Calcium deposits that collect on the optic nerve or the ganglia are cataracts. Loss of vision, glaucoma, and macular degeneration are symptoms of the same disease pathway.

Acid pH Plays A Role In Morning Sickness

When a woman gets pregnant, the fetus takes priority, drawing all the necessary alkaline minerals. Babies are born with the highest alkalinity. This means that while the mother is sleeping, she loses alkaline minerals, creating blood acidity. This phenomenon is known as morning sickness. By eating an alkaline diet and drinking alkaline beverages morning sickness will disappear.

The Life of The Flesh Is In The Blood

The Bible tells us that the life of the flesh is in the blood (Lev. 17:11). Without blood continuously pumping through our entire circulatory network every second of every day, we'd be dead. Scientifically we know that a constant battle to maintain balanced pH is taking place both within and out of our cells, our body fluids, and our blood at all times. If we take care of our body and feed it the proper nutrition, its pH levels take care of themselves, as automatically as the heart pumps blood.

By ingesting and exposing ourselves to an array of toxic acids that contaminate the blood we're disrupting our pH balance and destroying our health in the process. Knowing the important role pH plays in the blood, it's disturbing to see so many people abusing themselves by contaminating their bodies and blood with an overabundance of acidic compounds. Just look at some of the toxic acids people are putting into their bodies on a regular basis: alcohol, cigarettes, coffee, sugar, carbonated beverages, pharmaceuticals/antibiotics, red meat, and processed foods, just to list a few. These are all acid-producing, health-destroying substances that are poisonous to cellular health and, over time, will alter the body's critical pH levels.

Why is it that almost everything that tastes good and is bad for our health has a link to acidity? We are assaulted regularly with acid foods, acid beverages, acid rain, acid emotions (anger, fear, bitterness, stress, anxiety, etc.), acid pharmaceuticals, acid recreational drugs (cocaine, heroine, ecstasy, LSD, etc.), acid music, acid pesticides, acid herbicides, acid fungicides, acid industrial products, acid exhaust (cars, planes, etc.), acid based petroleum chemicals, *ad infinitum*. Is it possible that some kind of spiritual warfare is connected to this acidic assault upon us? It sure makes one wonder, especially when we understand that almost everything given to us by our Creator in its natural state has an alkalizing effect on the body and works to keep us in balance.

Conclusion

The battle between life and death and humanity's struggle with sickness is over pH. This is not a complicated issue to understand. As long as the body has sufficient alkaline potential from a well balanced diet and all of its elimination routes are open, cell-damaging acids can be safely neutralized and excreted from the body before cellular damage takes place. If we habitually consume fresh, organic, high alkaline-forming fruits, vegetables, nuts, seeds and legumes grown on rich topsoil, avoiding, as much as humanly possible the "acid landmines" of our modern civilization, we can properly alkalize the body and stay healthy.

The time is ripe for a paradigm shift to intelligent self-care, to greater consciousness of the divine mechanisms behind God's magnificent, self-healing system. We need a new level of understanding about the body's own inherent, innate and unquestionable ability to heal itself. It is time for a real and widespread wake-up call about the insidious enemies of self-healing; armored with a new awareness about the true cause – and cure – for ALL disease.

When our blood contains living nutrients, our body's cell metabolism and pH are in proper balance. When our cells are properly nourished, hydrated, and oxygenated, it is virtually impossible for us to become unwitting victims of illness and "disease." So the question is: Are you choosing **Death** through continually living in an acid environment, pursuing an acid lifestyle, or are you choosing *Life* by following a balanced lifestyle and nature's simple, yet exceedingly profound formula of alkalinity? The choice is up to each one of us.

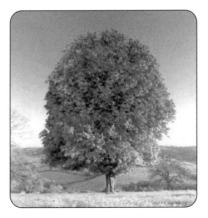

Tree of life

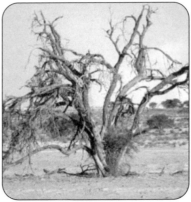

Tree of knowledge of good and evil (death)

PART II
Q & A

CRUSADOR Health Magazine Editor Greg Ciola Interviews Cutting-Edge Nutritional Scientist Gary Tunsky On The Important Role pH Plays In Optimum Health

"Bless the LORD, O my soul, and forget not all his benefits: Who forgiveth all thine iniquities; who healeth all thy diseases." **(Psalm 103:2-3)**

Gary Tunsky is a top nutritional scientist with a gifted ability to explain in eloquent detail how the body's cells function, what they require to stay healthy, and the critical role pH plays in this life process. A genius at connecting the dots and showing the whole picture of how and why blood and cells become acidic, Tunsky is quick to point out that what you think, drink, eat, breathe or bathe in either nourishes the blood and your body's 100 trillion cells with life force, or contaminates them, bringing disease and premature death.

As a nutritional scientist and disease consultant to thousands of patients, Tunsky's pioneering research has led him to conclude that most health problems, whether metabolic, degenerative, or autoimmune, are intricately linked to an excessively acidic cellular condition in the body. This means that the body's cells, tissues, and fluids are pH imbalanced and the blood is compensating by pulling alkalizing minerals (*i.e. calcium, potassium, magnesium, etc.*) from other areas of the body in order to maintain homeostasis at the blood and cellular level.

Tunsky is very critical of Western medicine and points out its colossal failure in understanding the intricate link between pH balance in the cells, tissues, and blood and a high state of health. Sadly, there are virtually no treatment modalities in Western medicine's toolbox that work within nature's boundaries to help alkalize your pH or modulate cell processes and immunity.

We all have the freedom to make our own choices about our health. This is our Constitutional, as well as our Divine right. We cannot allow ourselves – either through ignorance of health and/or lack of responsibility – to be manipulated by the medical establishment. Its primary interests revolve around ever-expanding drug profits from symptom suppression, instead of getting to the root cause of the problem: helping people regain their health. To do this ourselves we need accurate information so we can make decisions that lead us onto the path of health and long life, instead of into disease and premature death. The responsibility is up to you, me, each one of us. With an epidemic of health problems in the world today, we must become self-educated, informed health advocates because chances are most doctors are not going to have the answers we're looking for.

Let's take a brief microscopic look at the umbrella term "health-care-system." The U.S. has a so-called health care system that has nothing to do with the promotion of health. Those who run this system do not care about your health, and it's far from being a system. It's a fragmented patchwork of procedure-oriented services that are meshed in a voluminous trail of paper payments, with little relevance to community-based needs. This misdirected, disease-managed non-care system of symptom suppression demands more and more treatment at higher and higher costs. If they cared at all, you'd be treated like a human, not like a number resembling, quite frankly, the ear tags on a cattle herd.

If doctors had all the answers to our health problems, they would be curing most of the maladies people are suffering from today, without forcefully drugging over 60% of the population with toxic pharmaceuticals for the rest of their lives. That's why they call it "Practicing Medicine!" You're the guinea pig. Doctors are trained in "sick care" not health care. We actually have sick care insurance, not health care insurance. In other words, first you get sick; then they care if you have insurance.

Gary, you gave readers an extensive amount of information in Part I "The Battle For Health Is Over pH." In this interview I'd like to go into more detail, so that most of the questions people have on pH are answered. Let me begin by asking you how you can do a simple test at home to check your pH levels?

There's a fairly inexpensive roll of litmus paper that's available in many drug, health and natural food stores that can easily and rapidly test a person's urine or saliva. All you do is tear off an inch or so from the roll and dip it into saliva or urine. As soon as the paper is wet, the color changes within a range of shades, depending on your pH reading. A color chart comes with the roll, so you'll be able to match your sample to identify what your pH reading is. Generally the chart can measure pH levels between the ranges of 4.5 and 8.5. It's very simple.

What's the best time to check your pH levels?

I recommend testing your pH first thing in the morning when you wake up and once again right before you go to bed, as long as you haven't had anything to eat or drink for several hours to avoid false readings. It's best to check your pH levels at least twice a day. It's also very important to get a note pad and write down your readings each time to document the results so you can go back and see what kind of changes are occurring. I find that people who keep a record of these measurements with dates and times do much better on the program. Once they start seeing their pH levels change, they become much more enthusiastic knowing that they're making progress.

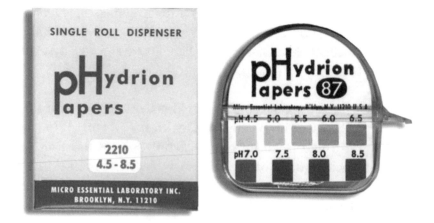

If not available in your area, pH litmus paper can be obtained through **CRUSADOR** by calling 1-800-593-6273.

Is it better to check your saliva or your urine, or should you check both?

You should check both. You want to check the saliva as an indicator of tissue and cell pH, and the urine as a measure of kidney excretion capability. You'll find that there will be a variance between the two and initially you want to see this. For the most part, you will see more acidity in the urine than you will in the saliva. This means that your internal detox systems, your kidneys and liver, are working to expel acid wastes from the body.

Your liver, lymphatic system, and kidneys are your primary blood-filtering systems. Acidic urine is an indication of acid waste residues coming out of the tissues. As excess acids get picked up from the cells and tissues, they are dumped into the blood and eventually filter through the kidneys for excretion. Once you go through a detox program, change your diet, and begin feeding1 your body alkaline foods and beverages, you should see the urine and saliva pH come pretty close to matching, however, your saliva should be slightly more alkaline than your urine.

What's the ideal pH range we should be striving to achieve?

With saliva, you should be aiming for a reading in the range of 7.0 to 7.5 pH. Most people are running between 5.5 and 6.5 pH. With urine, after a detox program and diet change, the ideal number is between 6.7 to 7.0 pH. I find many of my patients running acidic between a 4.5 and 6.0 pH in their urine. It's no wonder that the U.S. has an epidemic of viral and bacterial infections – and cancer. This pH range is a perfect breeding ground for anaerobic pathogens. After initiating a diet change, along with a comprehensive detox program, your pH levels should adjust to normal rather quickly.

What about checking your blood pH, can this be done at home?

No. This can only be done in the hospital. A doctor or nurse has to take an arterial blood draw and do a specific pH test called an ABG (Arterial Blood Gas). Generally this is done in emergency situations, if you're hemorrhaging from a serious car accident, undergoing anesthesia, or suffering from what is called metabolic or respiratory acidosis. Blood pH falls within a very narrow window, registering in the range of 7.30 to 7.45.

Do you ever recommend people to have their blood pH levels checked?

Only if my patients are in a life-threatening situation. The blood is usually the last place where you'll be able to detect a pH imbalance. Since blood is the body's life force, any slight variation in your pH levels could be very serious. The way your body regulates pH is similar to the way it regulates body temperature. Any variance up or down is usually a sign that something is wrong. The body has a very intelligent, built-in thermostat that knows precisely how to maintain a very tight pH range in the blood. A slight variation in your blood pH could result in death very quickly. This is why your body will pull alkaline potential (i.e. minerals, enzymes, amino acids, etc.) from your bones, joints, teeth, muscles and tissues into the blood to buffer acids. I call this the body's built-in "compensatory mechanism."

Is it true that lemons and limes can help regulate pH levels even though they are acidic fruits?

Yes. It's very interesting, and one of the amazing mysteries of nature. Both of these fruits can assist in balancing your pH. Although they are both acidic *in vitro* or *outside* the body, they actually become alkaline *invivo* or *inside* the body. Lemons and limes contain high amounts of bioavailable ionic calcium, mag-

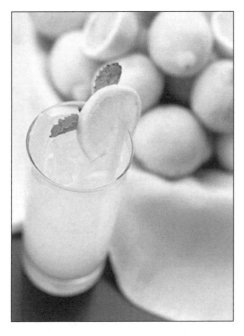

nesium and potassium – three alkaline minerals needed by the body to neutralize acids and regulate pH. As a result of poor diet and improper farming methods, many of us fail to get the correct kind and/or amount of minerals required and subsequently, suffer from terrible mineral deficiencies. Not only are we not getting adequate amounts of minerals from our daily diet, but also the body is depleting them faster than it can replace its reserves, which literally drains the mineral bank account. When this account finally goes bankrupt, disease will set in because the body has no other resources with which to neutralize the acids that are poisoning the tissues and cells.

I recommend that several times throughout the day you squeeze a fresh lemon or lime into 16-32 ounces of water and drink it. Make sure you don't use the processed concentrate that comes in a bottle – you want the freshest organic fruit possible. Drink this lemon/lime water instead of filling your body with acid producing soda pop and other toxic beverages. If you do, you'll be amazed at the impact this has on your kidney function, pH levels, and your overall health in just a matter of days.

There are other fruits, vegetables, nuts, grains and seeds that are naturally acidic, but once ingested work to alkalize the body.

Yes, this is true. If you were to look at a food chart, you

would notice an extensive number of foods that fall into the acidic category. I don't want readers to misconstrue what I'm saying, though. You don't want to avoid all acids, just all the manmade acids that come from packaged, bottled, canned, or processed foods and beverages. There's a big difference between these and fresh, whole, organic foods. There are really two kinds of acids: life-less enzyme-defi-cient acids from man-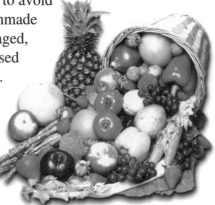made/processed foods or beneficial acids from nature. Fresh, live lemons and limes are good examples. Naturally occurring acids from raw, living foods can be alkaline forming, affecting the body in a positive way.

All food, once digested and processed, leaves an ash residue. This ash residue can have a much different pH than the actual pH of the food before it was eaten. The minerals present usually determine its value. Obviously your diet should consist of a high proportion of alkaline foods. However, you can't just survive on 100% alkaline foods alone, you have to balance your diet with natural acids to ensure proper pH in the stomach and other bodily fluids.

How much water should someone drink in a day to maintain optimum health and flush out acids?

There are many differing views within the alternative health field about how much water people need on a daily basis. Proper hydration of the cells is an important component to any health program. In my practice, I recommend a 1/2 oz. of water per pound of bodyweight, which seems to work very well with

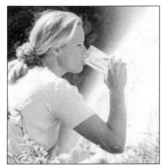

my patients. This means, for example, that if you weigh 160 pounds, you should drink at least 80 oz., or about ten 8 oz. glasses of water a day.

What kind of water do you recommend for drinking?

I have found that drinking alkaline water is the quickest and most effective way to change the body's pH and reverse acidosis, dehydration, and free radical damage. Alkaline water will hydrate, detoxify, and oxygenate your body's cells and act as a liquid antioxidant to neutralize harmful free radicals. There are two ways to obtain alkaline water. One is to purchase some of the bottled waters on the market that have a pH value above 7.5. Two of the better ones are Fiji and Trinity water. Fiji water has a natural pH of 7.5 and Trinity water has a pH of 9.6.

The other way to obtain alkaline water is to make it yourself. You can do this by purchasing a good water ionizer that you hook up to your sink faucet. The way a water ionizer works is two-fold. First, tap water is brought into the machine and run through a filter to remove most of the chemicals that don't belong there. Then the water is run through an electrolysis process containing a positive and negative conductor inside the machine. The result of this electrolysis process is separation and concentration of alkaline and acidic minerals. The alkaline minerals are pulled to one side and used to alter the pH of the water while the acidic minerals are safely removed from an exit hose. During this separation process the cluster size of the water is reduced, making it a "wetter water" that will hydrate the cells much better. This is where the terms "restructured" or "clustered" water come from. The electrolysis process also puts negative hydrogen ions into the water making it a powerful antioxidant within the body. There are numerous water ionizers on the market. I have found the Japanese units to be the best because they rarely break down.

If you can't obtain alkaline water I must caution everyone to be extremely suspect of the bottled water business. It's a very deceptive industry. After running tests on many of the major bottled waters on the market, I discovered that they are almost all acidic and still contain chemicals.

I do not recommend reverse osmosis water even though it takes the chemicals out of tap water because it generally runs between 4.0 and 5.0 pH, which is extremely acidic. Some spring waters are good but I have found that many of them are acidic too. One of the only spring waters that I've found to be consistently alkaline is Evian water. Acid rain deposits have ruined a lot of spring water and well water. If you know that the spring water you're getting comes from a reliable source and the pH is above 7.0 I think this is a fairly good alternative.

With regard to distilled water, you need to be careful if you use it on a regular basis because it has no bioavailable minerals and no electrical resonance properties. I have also discovered that distilled water runs between 5.0 and 5.5 pH. If you drink distilled water regularly you need to supplement your diet with plant-based ionic minerals to replace the electrolytes. In my opinion, distilled water is excellent to use for short periods of time because it's a powerful chelator that helps pull heavy metals and toxins out of the body. However, over long periods of time it has the potential to leach valuable minerals from your body, which could lead to problems down the road. You definitely want to stay away from drinking tap water unless it's properly filtered. It's full of cancer causing contaminants such as fluoride, chlorine, bromide, arsenic, lead, and other toxic chemicals.

Is it unhealthy to drink too much water?

This is very difficult to do. You would have to drink gallons to overdose, so to speak. Drinking water in large amounts for very short periods of time is recommended for correcting dehydration, replacing fluid from excessive exercise, or for fasting or cleansing. Otherwise, follow my advice of 1/2 ounce of water per pound of bodyweight.

Excessive urination is a sign that your body is attempting to eliminate the inorganic minerals and toxins present in the water that it cannot use. However, without an abundance of cell hydrating water your body's cells cannot function properly. Our bodies are over 70% water and most people are severely dehydrated, especially from drinking soda, coffee, alcohol and sugar/sodium-laden drinks regularly.

Again, it's very important to get your minerals from living whole foods, especially green foods. It's also important to supplement your diet with a high quality plant-derived liquid ionic mineral product. Large quantities of high quality water like Narawa will not make you urinate as frequently because the water is being efficiently utilized at the cellular level.

Once someone begins following an alkaline-based program, how quickly can they expect to see their pH levels change?

You should see your pH levels start to change in a matter of days if you follow through with the necessary treatment protocols, which I've outlined the **Seven "ATIONS" of treatment**. However, it can take weeks or even a few months to get your pH levels to a stable, balanced range required for re-establishing a high degree of health. There are many contributing factors and each patient is different. My **7-7-7 Program of Perfect Health** consists of:

The Seven "ATIONS" of Treatment for pH Imbalance and Cellular Malfunction

1.) DetoxificATION (colon, liver, gall bladder, kidneys, lymphatic system, blood)
2.) De-AcidificATION
3.) OxygenATION
4.) Nutritional AssimilATION
5.) Immune System ModulATION
6.) Full Body CirculATION (blood & lymph)
7.) Hormone ModulATION (estrogen, testosterone, thyroxin, progesterone)

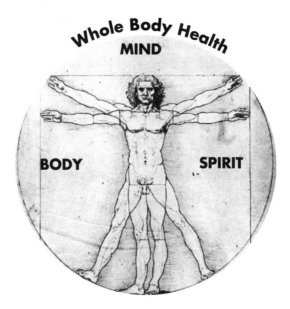

Whole Body Health
MIND
BODY
SPIRIT

The Seven "ATIONS" Of Cellular Insufficiencies

1.) Insufficient Respir**ATION** (oxygenation)
2.) Insufficient Hydr**ATION**
3.) Insufficient Toxin Elimin**ATION**
4.) Insufficient Immuniz**ATION**
5.) Insufficient Circul**ATION**
6.) Insufficient Communic**ATION**
7.) Insufficient Vibr**ATION** (energy or cell resonance)

The Seven "ATIONS" of Detoxification

1.) Increase Perspir**ATION** (sweating)
2.) Enhance Bowel Elimin**ATION** (colon cleanse)
3.) Increase Urin**ATION** (kidneys/bladder)
4.) Enhance Chel**ATION** (respiration/oxidation of heavy metals: i.e. cadmium, lead, aluminum, mercury)
5.) Increase Circul**ATION** (lymph & blood)

6.)   Enhance FiltrATION (liver, kidney and lymph-nodes)

7.)   Enhance MeditATION (to remove emotional and spiritual toxins)

Is it possible to have balanced pH and still be sick?

This is very rare, but possible. If this occurs, it could be due to emotional disturbances. There is an underlying emotional component to illness. Anger, bitterness, resentment, hatred, depression, and unforgiveness, which I call toxic emotions, are all negative and potentially damaging to health.

If someone is following the perfect pH-regulating program and they don't notice their pH levels modifying toward an alkaline range within a reasonable period of time, what would you recommend?

In this case I would tell them to incorporate a major detox-ification plan to unclog their filtering systems and support their digestion with enzymes. It's more than likely an indication that their liver is still backed up, their kidneys are clogged, their colon is full of waste, or their hormones and stomach enzymes are out of balance. They're probably not sweating enough to remove acid wastes either. It's vitally important for all of the elimination routes, including the lymphatic system, to be clear and function-ing simultaneously.

Your skin is a major acid eliminator. The skin is basically your third kidney because it removes up to one third of the toxins from your body. The kidneys, skin and lungs are the biggest out-lets for expelling uric, lactic, and carbonic acids along with acetyl acid which comes from alcohol.

Increasing your respiration and circulation through aer-obic exercises, massage, and/or weight resistance training is important. Carbon dioxide is a gaseous form of acid waste. We get rid of 300% more acid wastes through breathing out CO_2 than by any other way. Breathing in high amounts of oxygen and expelling CO_2 is one of the fastest ways to change pH. The more oxygen you breathe, the more carbon dioxide is expelled.

How many times a week should someone exercise?

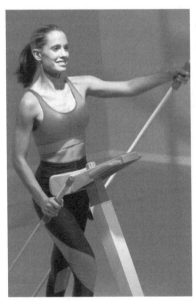

I recommend a good blend of aerobic and weight resistance exercise, at least three days a week for forty or more minutes at a time. Four to five days a week is optimal. Aerobic exercise increases lymph flow. The lymphatic system is a major factor in removing acids from the cells, but lymph nodes do not pump on their own, like the heart, they need to be manually pumped through exercise. When you focus and work on the muscles, your body composition of fat to muscle ratio changes and your metabolic rate increases.

What are some effective nutritional supplements people can take to help alkalize their body?

The most powerful alkalizing foods on the planet are the ones that are highest in chlorophyll. You just can't beat the nutritious, cell-restoring potential of green foods such as wheat, barley, kamut, alfalfa, and oat grasses along with spirulina and chlorella. They are thousands of times more powerful than ordinary green vegetables, because they are super concentrated in chlorophyll, alkaline minerals, rare trace minerals, vitamins, phyto-nutrients, and enzymes.

It's imperative that you use one or more of these potent green foods on a daily basis. They are available in convenient powder forms at many health food stores. Make sure that whatever product you use states that it's 100% organic, making it free of all pesticides and herbicides.

I also recommend other highly alkalizing supplements such as ionic minerals, oxygen drops, oxygen colon cleansers, pH water, detoxifying herbs, cayenne pepper, garlic, enzymes, aloe vera juice or gel, a high quality whole food multi-vitamin and mineral formula, organic herbal teas, and probiotics for re-establishing gut flora.

What can you tell us about the mineral cesium? A few network marketing companies are promoting it as a cellular pH regulator. Apparently this is a mineral that can enter the cell and change the pH internally.

I've heard the claims that cesium has the ability to enter the cell through osmosis and kick up the cellular pH internally instead of externally. I've never used cesium with any of my patients because I feel that it's not cost effective and potentially dangerous. There are much more economical ways of increasing your cellular pH than paying a hundred bucks a vial.

Cesium is an isolate and can become very toxic with long-term use. Any metal in large doses throws off homeostasis. We should not be focused on one mineral supplement as the silver bullet solution to fixing pH imbalances. We need a full-spectrum blend of minerals derived from plant life to restore cellular homeostasis. In my opinion, cesium is much too dangerous to take on a long-term basis because it severely depletes potassium from the cells, which could put a person at risk for muscle cramps and cardiac arrest.

What about coral calcium? This has become one of the biggest products ever to hit the supplement market. Is there any truth to coral calcium changing pH?

I find coral calcium to be just another marketing scam perpetrated by greedy supplement manufacturers. Some naturopathic doctors are claiming success with coral calcium, but they are not considering the long-term dangers and consequences. I find it very hard to believe the outrageous claims about coral calcium, since it's being sourced from dead, inorganic coral polyps that have degenerated into sand. This is basically no different than scooping up dirt or sand from your backyard. The body needs living minerals coming from living foods.

Taking high amounts of *any* calcium supplement can change pH levels in the saliva because calcium is a very alkaline mineral. Even calcium carbonate from chalkboard chalk will do that. But is this calcium getting into the cells? In my scientific opinion, probably not. And if it isn't, where is it being deposited – in the arteries, kidneys, eyes, heels, joints, gall ducts? How is the body filtering out the excess, unavailable calcium?

Chemically speaking, coral calcium is almost entirely calcium carbonate, which has never been proven to be a beneficial mineral for cellular health. It can't be utilized any more than drinking salt water can quench your thirst. Coral calcium may help people with heartburn and indigestion, just like most antacids on the market. The sad part, however, is that people take coral calcium, see their pH levels changing on the litmus paper, and then automatically assume it's doing something good for them. If we were to believe the marketing hype put out by the promoters of coral calcium, most diseases would be cured in a matter of a few months or even weeks. We're not seeing that kind of success with coral calcium. I think time will tell whether it is a beneficial supplement, but I say: BUYER BEWARE.

Is there a good time to eat for optimum pH balancing?

You need to eat small meals frequently throughout the day. Every three to four hours is ideal, if you can do it, but no more than 400 to 500 calories per meal. You should never eat late at night. Stop eating after 7:00 pm, if you can. This gives your body time to rest and digest food properly. I also recommend using a high-quality, plant-based enzyme supplement with each meal to help break down and digest your foods.

At night you should drink plenty of water with lemon or lime, or herbal teas and fresh vegetable juices, which are also very alkalizing and nutritionally beneficial. If you're one of those that must eat late at night, have a piece of low glycemic fruit or a vegetable salad.

What's the correct acid/alkaline ratio of foods people should be consuming?

From all the research I've done and from first hand experience, I find that a balance of 80% alkaline and 20% acid works best. I don't want people to think that all acids are bad. There are fluids and enzymes in the body that thrive and function on a sub-acid or acid pH. For example, hydrochloric acid in your stomach has a pH value of less than 1.0. Your body needs a balanced blend of acid and alkaline substances.

The acid foods I recommend to make up this 20% are living, whole foods in a pure natural state, such as organic eggs and sprouted grains. Definitely not the manmade, poisonous acid "foods" created in the laboratory. Many people today are consuming a diet that's 80% acid and 20% alkaline, with a fountain of acid coming from sugar, white flour, soda, coffee, alcohol, bottled fruit juices, fried foods and unclean meats such as pork and shellfish. Though it's virtually impossible to consume a diet that's 100% alkaline, an overly alkaline diet can bring your pH too high, which is not healthy either. It's balance that we're after.

Can your tongue be a good indicator of excess acids in the body, and if so, what should someone look for?

The feel of your mouth can definitely be a good indicator of your pH. Generally, an acidic mouth will feel dry and dirty, as though your teeth and tongue need to be brushed. The tongue may get a whitish film on it, which is an indicator of a fungal condition called Thrush. Yeast, bacteria and viruses grow in an acid medium, clinging to the tongue and teeth as food sources. With a properly balanced pH (7.0-7.5), saliva is slightly alkaline, and yeast, fungal forms, bacteria and viruses have a very difficult time surviving. Your mouth and teeth will feel clean, even after you eat, and your tongue will also have a healthy pinkish tone to it.

Bad breath or halitosis goes hand in hand with an acidic pH. Everyone I have ever consulted with who has a problem with bad breath had acidic pH. When the pH levels rise to an alkaline state, bad breath disappears, along with the anaerobic pathogens that cause gingivitis and periodontal disease. This is also why a good organic toothbrush, tongue scraper, and fluoride-free, tooth-cleansing agents are so important. They help scrub off bacteria, viruses and fungal forms from your teeth and tongue.

What about Essential Fatty Acids? Many health conscious consumers are convinced that we need them in our diet. What role do they play in regulating pH?

The whole subject of essential fatty acids (EFA's) would require a book in and of itself to properly explain their role in nutrition and health, so let me do my best to sum it up briefly. A major factor interfering with cell health and pH is toxic oils, hydrogenated fats, and *transfats*. Americans are literally killing themselves by consuming thousands of foods full of these toxic oils on a regular basis.

EFA's are an important component in cell membranes. The cell membrane surrounds the cell and controls what enters and exits the cell, protecting the cell. When toxic oils and hydrogenated fats are consumed, they can coat the cell membrane, making them hard like stone, completely disrupting the respiration process of the cell. The effect that improper oils has on the cells and arteries is analogous to me sticking a plastic bag over your head and expecting you to breathe. It wouldn't take long for you to die from asphyxiation. A similar process occurs at the cel-

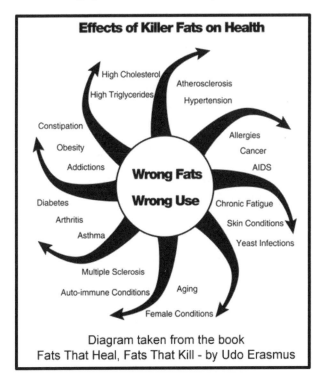

Effects of Killer Fats on Health

High Cholesterol
High Triglycerides
Atherosclerosis
Hypertension
Constipation
Obesity
Addictions
Allergies
Cancer
AIDS
Wrong Fats
Wrong Use
Diabetes
Arthritis
Asthma
Chronic Fatigue
Skin Conditions
Yeast Infections
Multiple Sclerosis
Auto-immune Conditions
Aging
Female Conditions

Diagram taken from the book
Fats That Heal, Fats That Kill - by Udo Erasmus

lular level with these solidifying toxic fats. The only difference is that you have 100 trillion cells in your body and the process takes longer.

When cell membranes are composed of polyunsaturated fatty acids, they are flexible and elastic. The scientific research available on the role the proper-ratio of Omega 3's, 6's, and 9's play in health is remarkable. Essential fatty acids are responsible for transporting oxygen and nutrients from the bloodstream into the cells. Without the right blend of these important oils in your diet, all cell processes will be disrupted, including pH balance.

First and foremost, it's absolutely critical to completely eliminate all forms of toxic oils, including hydrogenated, partially-hydrogenated, and *transfats* from your diet. Secondly, it's imperative that you take a high quality supplement from a health food store with the right blend of essential fatty acids. There are many from which to choose. An excellent book to learn more about the important role essential fatty acids play in health is Udo Erasmus' **Fats That Heal, Fats That Kill.**

How about sugar? Do we need to avoid it altogether or is there a safe amount we can eat?

Regardless of the client, one of the first things I recommend is to completely eliminate all forms of sugar. There are no exceptions. Sugar is one of the most acidifying substances in the world. Not only will it decimate your pH balance, it's the primary food source for the microorganisms that thrive in an acidic pH, including cancer cells. Feeding sugar to any bacteria, virus, fungus or parasite is like throwing gasoline on a fire. It's their number one favorite energy source. Until you shut off sugar consumption, you'll never be able to eliminate dangerous, health-crippling microorganisms or restore your pH.

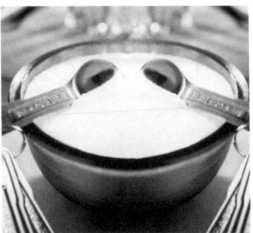

I've seen estimates that the average American consumes 175 lbs. of sugar per year. Sugar disrupts all body chemistry; severely weakens the immune system, and is implicated in over 100 health problems including diabetes, allergies, heart disease and obesity. For example, sugar upsets the balance of minerals, increases triglycerides, interferes with the absorption of calcium and magnesium, weakens eyesight and causes tooth decay. It even impairs the structure of DNA, causes free radicals, damages and over-stresses the pancreas, makes bones brittle, causes depression, and slows down the ability of the adrenals to function.

The problem is that people are addicted to sugar just like a drug, and it's very difficult to get them to completely eliminate this highly acidic substance from their diet. Sugar can come from a number of different sources and unless you're aware of the landmines to avoid, it's still possible to overwhelm your system with sugar without even knowing it. For starters, all table sugar and all packaged goods that list sugar, cane juice, beet sugar, fructose, corn syrup, maltodextrin, high fructose corn syrup, barley malt, or rice syrup must be avoided at all costs.

The next sugar assault comes from carbohydrates. Now, I'm not saying that all carbohydrates are bad, but you need to understand that carbohydrates quickly convert to sugar or glucose in the body. Due to the high glycemic index and lack of nutrients, almost all the carbohydrates in refined, processed foods are just as damaging to the body as straight table sugar. You should only be eating complex carbohydrates that come from whole foods the way nature gave them to us, proportionately balanced with protein, essential fatty acids, minerals, enzymes, and vitamins that work together in synergy to slow down glucose triggering for insulin release.

Some fruits and vegetables such as potatoes, beets, pineapple, and watermelon, once broken down, have too high of a sugar content and should be avoided initially if you're trying to restore your pH levels. Once your body's pH is in balance, it's okay to incorporate these fruits and vegetables back into your diet, but they should be eaten in small amounts. Many fruits like lemons, limes, and avocados and many vegetables with a low glycemic index, such as salad and all your green vegetables <u>do not</u> impact blood glucose levels negatively and are okay to eat in appropriate quantities. Dr Robert Young's books **The pH Miracle** and **Sick and Tired?: Reclaim Your Inner Terrain** along with Dr. Mercola's **Total Health Cookbook and Program** have some excellent recipes and lists of foods that will help you prepare healthy meals that won't negatively impact your glucose levels.

In "The Battle For Health Is Over pH" you mentioned that when you become acidic, your body pulls sodium bicarbonate into the blood from other areas of the body to neutralize acids. Can you drink sodium bicarbonate (baking soda) to change your pH levels?

You should never use this unless it's in a crisis situation. Sodium bicarbonate in common baking soda is a very high alkaline buffering agent. The problem is it destroys vitamins in the body and it's not a beneficial source of sodium to work at the cellular level. Sodium bicarbonate can change pH too fast. The only time I would ever even recommend drinking sodium bicarbonate is with the advice of a certified nutritionist or doctor in a crisis situation.

What about nutritional supplements? Are any of them a source of acids? If so, what should we look out for?

Many of the vitamins on the market are created synthetically, using carbon chain constructs and petroleum by-products, which are possible sources of unnatural acids and toxins. You should use vitamins and herbs that come from whole food complexes with the enzymes, amino acids, minerals, and phytonutrients in their natural state, allowing them to be utilized at the cellular level.

Be aware of the binders, fillers and excipients used during the encapsulation process as well. Things like magnesium stearate, stearic acid and glycerin are very common for binding tablets and filling capsules. If the label doesn't state that they come from vegetable sources, chances are pretty good that they come from rendered animal fats. These excipients can be acidifying to the body. Just check the label of any tablet or capsule you ingest, whether it's a vitamin or a pharmaceutical. Below the formula it should list "other ingredients" and this is where you'll see what they used. Your best bet is to look for whole food concentrated vitamins and green food blends that have natural vegetarian based binders and fillers. If it doesn't say whole food concentrate, chances are it's synthetic, and if it's synthetic, more than likely it's going to be rejected as foreign and have an acidifying effect on the body.

What role can fasting play in removing excess acids from the body?

Fasting with fresh vegetable juices is one of the quickest ways to remove acids from the body and correct pH imbalances. Vegetable juice fasting eliminates the poisons and toxins from your organs, tissues, cells, and glands that are contributing to your acidic condition. I am not a big fan of fasting with only water. A very toxic person can become sick by detoxifying too quickly with a strict water fast. This is commonly known as a Herxheimer reaction.

Start out with a vegetable juice fast before going on a complete water fast. During the first few days of your fast you should be showing acidic readings on the pH test strips in your urine and saliva. After this, these readings should modify towards an alkaline level. Building yourself up to be able to withstand a 7-10 day vegetable juice fast at least twice a year will go a long way toward keeping your system alkaline, cleansed, and balanced.

Can fragrant essential oils such as myrrh, frankincense, and spikenard help in any way to increase or alkalize pH?

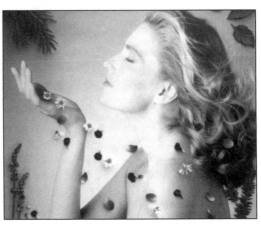

Absolutely. Essential oils are highly alkalizing because they are the blood of the plant. They have life force, which means that they have high frequency. Applied to the body, their high electromagnetic frequency helps to increase the life frequency resonance of the cell. Essential oils are also abundant in oxygen, one of the most powerful adjuncts for neutralizing acids and increasing pH. Their high medicinal value from terpenes and sesquiterpene compounds give them antibacterial, antiviral, antifungal, antiseptic and anti-tumor properties.

Can people experience these benefits by applying oils topically or is there another way to utilize essential oils?

You can apply them topically, breathe them through a diffuser (aromatherapy), or consume them internally in very small amounts of juice or water. Ideally, for best results, you should rub the oils on your feet at the junctures of powerful acupuncture meridians. When you breathe the oils diffused in the air through

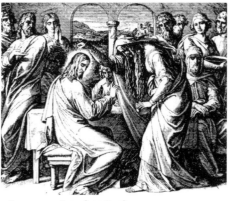
**Jesus anointed at Bethany
(Matthew 26:6-7)**

aromatherapy, the high frequency oxygen molecules go quickly through the olfactory sensory nerves directly to the brain (medulla) and into the bloodstream, where they are absorbed into the cells within 20 minutes. I am truly amazed at the powerful results I have seen with essential oils, God's healing medicines used for thousands of years in the Bible.

What about sunlight, can it help to balance pH and is it necessary for whole body health?

Sunlight plays a very important role in overall health, including balancing pH. Despite all the advice from the "so-called" experts that say sunlight is bad for you, photon rays from the sun are necessary for healthy cellular output and division. Each spectrum of color has an energy frequency or life force that genetically codes the cells to resonate in harmony. These beneficial rays are absorbed through your skin and your retina. That's why I recommend that you don't use sunglasses or sun block when you're outside either. You need to absorb this rainbow of color and photon light through your eyes and skin for at least 15-20 minutes a day if possible without the use of artificial blocking agents. Without adequate sunlight plant life would die. The same is true for people. I would caution you to beware of most of the sun blocks on the market. Unless they contain 100% natural ingredients there's a good chance they have carcinogenic substances in them that can poison the body and potentially cause skin cancer.

A deficiency in antioxidants and essential fatty acids is a big factor in why the sun damages DNA. Without adequate supplies of antioxidants in the body too much exposure to sunlight will cause direct free radical damage by robbing electrons. This is why correcting nutritional deficiencies is so important. Millions of Americans suffer from a condition called mal-illumination from being stuck working long hours in a stuffy, stale environment that has synthetic lighting. This is extremely detrimental to your overall health, including your mental state. Depression can set in from minimal exposure to full-spectrum lighting. You also get vitamin D from the sun and other nutrients that your body cannot produce despite the experts who claim they can be obtained from diet. However, if you live in places like Arizona, Texas and Florida, I would caution you to not get your daily exposure of sunlight during the peak hours of the day. The 15-20 minutes I recommend are in the morning or later in the afternoon when your chances of getting burned are virtually impossible.

What effect does chlorinated shower water have on the body's pH?

It has a very damaging effect. Chlorine and other water chemical disinfectants are acidic gases, creating aerosolized toxic vapors. When you take a hot shower, all of your pores open up and become a sponge for whatever chemicals are in the water. These toxic chemicals can go straight into your blood, organs, tissues, and cells, forcing your body to pull alkaline minerals from the bones, joints, teeth and other areas of the body to neutralize these acids.

These chemicals are especially harmful to your lungs, since you breathe these chemical vapors in first. The lungs are a conduit to the blood, so everything you breathe eventually passes into your bloodstream. Once in the bloodstream, your liver and kidneys have to filter these chemicals out. A perfect alkaline/acid base diet can literally be destroyed in a ten-minute shower. If you're serious about your health and raising your pH, then I strongly recommend you purchase a high quality shower filter that can take most of these acid poisons out of your water.

One of the best shower filters on the market for filtering toxins out of your water is made by **WaterWise**. It's called the **ShowerWise Filtration System**. If not available in your area they're available through *CRUSADOR* by calling 1-800-593-6273. They retail for $79.

What about most of the commercial soaps, shampoos, deodorants, creams, toothpastes, mouthwash, etc.?

Most commercial soaps, cosmetic and other personal hygiene products contain dangerous acidic chemicals. Just look on the back of the labels. You can't even pronounce many of these chemicals, let alone assimilate them. When applied directly to your body, these detrimental agents absorb through your pores or scalp into your blood, tissues, organs and cells, just like chemical vapors from your shower.

Your skin is your largest elimination organ for acids. Instead of being expelled as wastes, chemicals in commercial beauty and skin care products are actually absorbed like a sponge. Take antiperspirants, for example. Sweating produces acid wastes under your armpits. Applying antiperspirant shuts down an acid release mechanism, pushing these wastes back into the lymph nodes. This can increase the

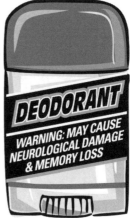

risk of breast cancer and suppress the immune system.

Inorganic commercial toothpastes and mouthwashes are also acidic and hazardous. Caustic chemicals like the sodium fluoride in these products get swallowed and absorbed into your bloodstream. You'd be amazed at what gets approved for use in cosmetics and toothpaste. Take a look at the back label of any fluoride-containing toothpaste. They warn you right on the packaging that it's a poison, yet it passes with FDA approval. **[Actual warning says: WARNING: As with all fluoride toothpastes, keep out of the reach of children under 6 years of age. If you accidentally swallow more than used for brushing, seek professional assistance or contact a Poison Control Center immediately.]** There are many fluoride-free alternatives in health food stores, but you still have to be careful because some of these poisons have crept into products that are sold there as well.

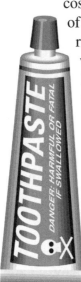

Don't be fooled by the word "natural" either. Make sure you learn more about this subject and read labels thoroughly to monitor what you're exposing yourself to. Many claim to be "natural" but this is largely a marketing term with no standards. You'll still find harmful acidic chemicals in products that claim to be natural.

Well Gary, it has been a pleasure hearing your thoughts on all these topics. Thank you for taking the time to thoroughly expound on these questions and enlighten our audience further. I'm sure that anyone reading this book will have a much better understanding of the whole subject of pH.

PART III

Pulling It All Together

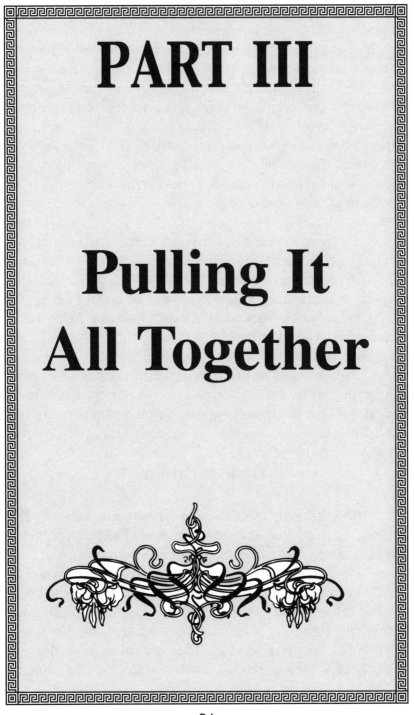

After learning about the importance of proper pH balance in the body and the role it plays in health, you may feel a bit overwhelmed when choosing a specific program to follow. It's impossible to market a one-size-fits-all program, since everyone's body is different and each one's state of health can vary so greatly. While there are specific sets of health protocols based on common denominators everyone should follow, you, yourself, may require other strategies or approaches depending upon the location of cellular malfunction, how your body responds, or how serious your health condition may be. Outlined below are some simple steps you can take to get started.

For more thorough and complete information on pH, you should purchase other reference materials and health books, especially books on preparing healthy meals and fully implementing detoxification. I highly recommend both of Dr. Robert O. Young's books, **Sick and Tired? Reclaim Your Inner Terrain** and **The pH Miracle**, as well as Hulda Clark's books, **The Cure For All Diseases** and **The Cure For All Cancers**. You should also seek out a reputable, holistically-oriented health practitioner in your area that practices integrative medicine, particularly if you have cancer or any other serious autoimmune or systemic disease.

Detoxification

The first thing recommended for anyone to balance pH is to undergo a complete 21-day detoxification program. Detoxification is the term used to describe the process your body goes through to get rid of toxins. When you take more toxins into your body than you can safely eliminate, excess toxins will store in your cells, tissues, organs, glands, and bones. Cleansing and detoxifying your body of unwanted acid wastes is the best way to begin correcting pH imbalances. There are at least eight different detoxification measures that should be undertaken to eliminate toxins from your entire body.

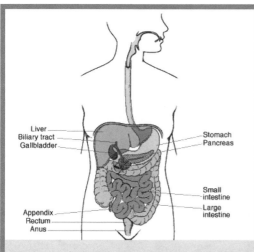

Liver
Biliary tract
Gallbladder
Appendix
Rectum
Anus
Stomach
Pancreas
Small intestine
Large intestine

Notice when looking at the following anatomy that the entire gastro-intestinal system and internal organs are intertwined as one complete unit. When one malfanctions, the entire system malfunctions.

1.) Colon Cleanse: The first area of the body one should detoxify is the colon. The reason for this is fairly obvious: A clogged and diseased colon is the first in line in the elimination system and can lead to the liver, kidneys, gall bladder and lymphatic system backing up with toxins. There are a number of effective ways to cleanse your colon.

a.) Oxygen colon cleansing supplements
b.) Home colonics/enemas
c.) Outpatient colonics at licensed clinics
d.) Coffee enemas
e.) Herbal laxatives
f.) High fiber/psyllium
g.) Rectal ozone treatments

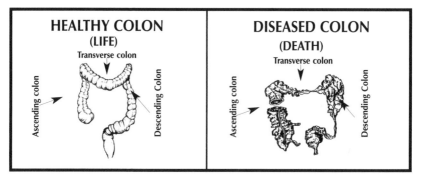

HEALTHY COLON
(LIFE)
Transverse colon
Ascending colon
Descending Colon

DISEASED COLON
(DEATH)
Transverse colon
Ascending colon
Descending Colon

2.) Liver Cleanse: The liver should be the second area of your body to detoxify. Most of the biochemical activity of detoxification takes place in the gastrointestinal system and liver. The liver is responsible for filtering toxic residues from the blood and transforming them into harmless, water soluble, biodegradable substances that can be filtered through the

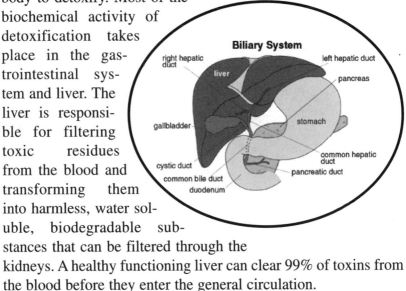

kidneys. A healthy functioning liver can clear 99% of toxins from the blood before they enter the general circulation.

There are many medicinal herbs and nutritional supplements that can help cleanse the liver and remove toxic compounds, including homeopathic remedies, coffee enemas, milk thistle, wormwood, and mushroom extracts. There are several different liver cleansing programs promoted in holistic medicine that are very effective. If you'd like to learn more about these specific cleanses, you can find them in Hulda Clark's book, **The Cure For All Diseases** and Burton Goldberg's well-known resource book, **Alternative Medicine**, **The Definitive Guide**.

3.) Kidney Cleanse: The kidneys play an extremely important role in pH balance and optimum health. After the colon and liver, it's best to focus on detoxifying and cleansing your kidneys. The kidneys are part of both the urinary and endocrine systems, performing numerous functions such as: eliminating metabolic waste, filtering the blood, producing hormones, regulating blood pressure, balancing electrolytes, balancing acid/alkaline levels. Kidneys are also responsible for vitamin D activation, prostaglandin synthesis, and erythrocyte production. There are many good herbs, nutritional supplements and homeopathic remedies available to effectively cleanse and detoxify your kidneys. One excellent thing you can do for your kidneys is to drink plenty of clean, mineral-rich water with fresh lemons or limes squeezed into it throughout the day on a regular basis. Both books mentioned in point 2 also have extensive information on kidney cleansing programs.

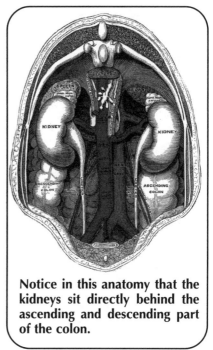

Notice in this anatomy that the kidneys sit directly behind the ascending and descending part of the colon.

4.) Lymphatic Cleanse: The lymphatic system plays an important role in pH balance because it is responsible for removing acidic wastes within and around the cells. Intricately linked to your immune system, it consists of lymph nodes, and the tonsils, spleen, and thymus. Lymph nodes are found primarily in the armpits, groin, breasts, and neck and are responsible for collecting lymphatic fluid. The tonsils, spleen, and thymus produce white blood cells known as lymphocytes to scavenge for toxins and microbes.

The lymphatic system does not have a pump like the heart to keep lymphatic fluid moving. Instead, it depends upon exercise, lymphatic massage, and other forms of compression to keep the system cleansed and operational. Pekana and Heel homeopathic remedies have been shown to be very effective in cleansing the lymphatic system. For more detailed information about the lymphatic system and cleansing options, see the book **Alternative Medicine, The Definitive Guide**.

5.) Gallbladder Cleanse: The gallbladder is an organ located directly under your liver. The liver uses bile to remove toxic substances from the blood. Bile goes first to the gallbladder until food arrives in the small intestine. Abnormal concentration of bile acids, cholesterol, and phospholipids in the bile can cause the formation of gallstones. Cleansing the gallbladder is often overlooked, but is another area of the body that should be addressed when it comes to detoxification. The books cited in point 2 above are also great resource materials for learning how to incorporate a gallbladder cleanse.

6.) Increased Perspiration (sweating): When most people focus on detoxification, they forget to include the skin as an area that should be addressed, as well. The skin is your body's largest organ. The skin sweats, breathes, and eliminates more cellular waste than the colon, liver, and kidneys combined. The bottom line is that you need to intervene and create a situation where your body sweats profusely for at least 30 minutes 3-4 days a week. The three most effective methods are exercise, steam sauna, and far infrared sauna.

7.) Chelation Therapy: Chelation therapy has proven to be one of the most effective ways to rid the body of heavy metals. Chelation agents bind to heavy metal toxins and excrete them through the skin, colon, and kidneys. Several different options available for chelation therapy are oral and IV chelation, mercury DMSA or DMPS, and suppository chelation with a product called Detoxamin. Calcium EDTA (not sodium EDTA), chlorella, garlic, and cilantro are also natural effective chelation agents. It would be best to seek out a chelation specialist in this field to explain the various techniques used.

8.) Emotional And Spiritual Cleanse: The two most neglected areas of research in disease epidemiology are the unseen levels of spirit and soul. In addition to physical toxins, there are emotional, as well as spiritual toxins, such as suppressed negative feelings and trauma from past experiences that become imbedded or held in pressure points and cells within the body. To fully establish and experience real health within the whole person, these toxins must also be cleansed. By removing the emotional toxins of anger, hatred, bitterness, stress, anxiety, unforgiveness, etc., and by purging the body of built up contaminants, you can allow the whole body to heal.

Increase Oxygenation

Oxygen deprivation at the blood and cellular levels is a major factor in disease, especially cancer. It is a *major* problem in an acidic body. Low oxygen levels allow microorganisms to breed and thrive. Almost every form of disease has its roots in some form of cellular respiratory problem where the blood is either not getting enough oxygen, or the cells aren't absorbing enough oxygen. In many cases it's a combination of the two. Oxygen has been called the breath of God and is known to be the most powerful cleansing and detoxification agent in the universe. Here are a few things you can do to increase your oxygen levels.

● **Start drinking freshly made vegetable juices** with chlorophyll-rich green foods (i.e. wheatgrass, barley, alfalfa, and/or oat grass, etc.) on a daily basis. Chemically, chlorophyll is virtually identical to hemoglobin and is a good blood builder and cellular oxygenator. Try to drink at

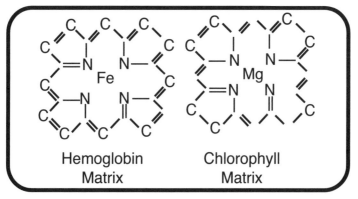

Hemoglobin
Matrix

Chlorophyll
Matrix

least 1 ounce a day of one or more of the above grasses, freshly juiced. Or use a good powdered supplement as a substitute.

- **Exercise more regularly**. Do some form of aerobic or anaerobic exercise for at least 20-30 minutes three to four times per week. This could include weight resistance training, walking, jogging, biking, swimming, stairmaster, spinning, martial arts, aerobics, etc.

- **Use deep breathing techniques**. There are many different breathing techniques that you can learn from books that specialize in this subject. All the major bookstores should have information available. One effective technique is to stand with your feet shoulder width apart, your hands on your hips, and your knees slightly bent. Take a deep breath through your nose until your lungs are filled to maximum capacity. With your head slightly up and your back slightly arched, slowly exhale through your mouth with your jaw closed and your tongue pressed against your front teeth. It should sound like you're letting the air out of a tire for about 20-30 seconds. You want pressure, so make sure you flex your abs or abdominal muscles when exhaling. Take 7-10 deep breaths like this and do it at least once a day.

- **Incorporate supplemental oxygen products** into your regimen like oxygen drops and food grade hydrogen peroxide that can be added to your water in small amounts.

- **Use exotic oxygenation techniques** available in alternative medicine clinics such as hyperbaric oxygen and the many forms of ozone/oxygen treatments.

- **Use a negative ion or ozone air purifier** in your home and office.

- **Use essential oils and aromatherapy**, which can carry oxygen deep into the lungs.

- **Use massage therapy and reflexology techniques** to stimulate blood flow and circulation.

Correct Nutritional Deficiencies
Enhance Nutritional Assimilation

Most people are suffering with nutritional deficiencies. Poor diets, poor quality supplements, and many environmental factors are delivering inadequate nutrition, keeping us from enjoying a high state of health. In order for nutritional deficiencies and imbalances to be corrected, you must first incorporate detoxification therapies. Otherwise, the body will not properly absorb or utilize the nutritional elements you feed it.

To begin, it's best to start feeding your body with those foods and beverages that bring life to it. Stop eating all of the lifeless, de-mineralized, devitalized, and dead, processed foods that only contribute to your body's breakdown. If you're eating dead foods that have been in a box, can, jar, package, freezer, or microwave, you are slowly digging your grave with your teeth. Once you feed the body proper nutrition, your pH levels will stabilize and come into balance very quickly. Here is a list of nutritional priorities to focus on. (See juicing recipes at the end of this section to help correct nutritional deficiencies)

1.) Vitamins: The best way to get your vitamins is from food. Life begets life, death begets death. You can't get life from dead foods. You need raw, whole food complexes for optimum nutrition, not synthetic multi-vitamin supplements that your body cannot utilize. Fresh, organic produce and fresh homemade fruit/vegetable juices are some of the best sources of natural vitamins. Green foods and bee pollen both contain high amounts of vitamins. If you feel you aren't getting enough raw fruits and vegetables for your daily vitamin requirements, you can supplement your diet with a good whole food multi-vitamin. Any reputable health food store can direct you to a high quality brand. Just be sure to specify that you want a vitamin made from 100% whole food.

2.) Minerals: Due to the high amount of processed foods grown on depleted soils that many people have been eating regularly for years, mineral deficiencies are at epidemic levels in this country. Most of your minerals should be obtained from raw, whole foods just like your vitamins. Minerals play an extremely important role in balancing pH. In addition to raw foods, many sea vegetables have a high, full-spectrum mineral content that is not only very beneficial, but noticeably uplifting and energizing.

You can also supplement your diet with minerals, but they should be in a liquid form that is either angstrom, ionic or nano particle size, never a tablet form. If you take a capsule, the minerals should be in a chelated form. This means that the mineral has been bonded to an amino acid or lipid so it will more easily enter the cell. Minerals are designed to be taken synergistically in combination, so do not take isolated mineral supplements. Be sure that if you supplement your diet with minerals, they are in a comprehensive blend.

3.) Enzymes: Enzymes are responsible for nearly every facet of life and are needed to help control all mental and physical functions. Enzymes are found in all living cells, including raw foods or those that are cooked at a temperature below 116 degrees. Enzymes transform minerals into alkaline detoxifying agents which combine with acidic cellular wastes and toxic settlements within the body, neutralizing them for elimination.

Enzymes, minerals, and vitamins all work together in synergy. It's very important to eat a diet containing at least 30-50% raw foods. Raw foods are bursting with living enzymes that are necessary for digestion and cellular health. There are many high quality digestive enzyme supplements on the market that can be used, as well. If you eat cooked food, it's a necessity that you take a full-spectrum plant-based enzyme supplement with each meal.

4.) Amino Acids/Lightweight Polypeptides: Amino acids are the building blocks that make up proteins. They are also the end products of protein digestion. Every living organism is composed of protein and every living cell in your body requires protein. The enzymes and hormones that catalyze and regulate all bodily processes are made of proteins, including those that maintain water balance and proper internal pH. Range-fed turkey, salmon, coldwater fish, organic eggs and egg yolks, nuts, lentils, various beans, and ionic-exchanged whey protein are the best sources of protein. If you're not getting enough amino acids in your diet, there are some excellent supplements to choose from at the health food store.

5.) Essential Fatty Acids (Omega 3's, 6's & 9's): EFA's are vital components of fats that work in conjunction with other nutrients in the body to prevent and reverse disease. Every meal you eat should include a serving of beneficial EFA's. The right amount of fats and oils in your diet can have a profound impact on your level of health. There are a variety of beneficial oils on the market such as flax, extra virgin olive, hemp, evening prim-rose, coconut and various seed oils. My favorite all around sup-plement is Udo's Oil from Flora. To learn more about this subject and what to look for, read the book, **Fats That Heal, Fats That Kill** by Udo Erasmus.

Modulate/Boost Your Immune System

The immune system plays a key role in the repair and maintenance of body tissues. Your immune system is the only defense that prevents you from being riddled with opportunistic infections, cancer, and a host of other chronic illnesses. You can't rejuvenate or repair the immune system with poisonous pharma-ceutical drugs or surgery. You can only modulate the immune sys-tem through natural methods. The immune system's surveillance barrier is an extremely important aspect to protect in order to restore health and prevent the onset of chronic health problems.

Enhancing the immune system means you don't just boost one or two components. There are actually 22 different instruments or components to the immune system including T-cells, B-cells, Natural Killer cells (NK cells), macrophages, lymphocytes, leukocytes, monocytes, interferon, gamma globulin, interleukin I, II, III, IV and other white blood cell components. All 22 must be supported simultaneously, orchestrated like a symphony or tuning in a piano, in order to restore or maintain optimum immunity. Here is a list of the more powerful immune enhancers/modulators being used in alternative medicine.

- **Colostrum:** This is the first fluid secreted by the mammary glands of mammalian mothers in the first days after giving birth. Contains high levels of protein and growth factors, as well as immune factors. Used around the world as one of the most powerful immune boosters known to man. The only colostrum you should use must state specifically that it's 100% from New Zealand cows. Outside of New Zealand it's very hard to guarantee that colostrum comes from cows that were grass fed and free of antibiotics, growth hormones and steroids.
- **Transfer Factors:** Tiny protein signaling molecules isolated from colostrum that serve as messengers for the immune system.
- **Olive Leaf Extract:** Fights all types of bacteria, viruses, fungi, and parasites and is good for virtually any infectious disease.
- **Royal Jelly:** Fed only to queen bees. Contains over 100 nutritional properties and has long been known to strengthen the immune system.
- **Pollen:** Plant pollen that bees harvest and pre-digest. Excellent for people with allergies, since it strengthens the immune system.
- **Propolis:** Resinous substance that bees derive from trees and mix with beeswax. Used as a health shield for the beehive, propolis is antibacterial, antiviral, antifungal, and antiseptic. Has been used for thousands of years as an

immune system booster.

- **Aloe Vera:** Contains high amounts of mucopolysaccha rides which kick in the immune modulators to fight off disease.
- **Homeopathic Remedies**
- **Mushroom Extracts (Shiitake, Reishi, D-Fraction Maitake):** Have excellent immune-boosting properties. Shiitake increases T-cell function, Reishi has anti-tumor properties, and Maitake enhances the activity of key immune cells known as T-helper cells or CD4 cells.
- **Echinacea:** Excellent herb for the immune system and the lymphatic system.
- **Acerola Berries/Vitamin C:** Helps prevent free radical damage and has antifungal and astringent properties.
- **Garlic:** Has antibacterial, antiviral, antifungal, and antiseptic properties and has long been used to fight off and prevent colds and infections.
- **Beta-1,3-Glucan:** Stimulates the activity of macrophages, immune cells that destroy debris, microorganisms, and abnormal cells by surrounding and digesting them.
- **Probiotics:** Rebuild intestinal flora, which is a front line defense for the body's immune system.

Balance/Modulate Your Hormones

As you age or when the body becomes too toxic, your hormones often become disrupted or stop functioning properly. Hormones affect virtually every bodily process and act upon all organs and systems. The subject of how to regulate your hormones through natural means and all the problems surrounding hormonal imbalances would require an entire book. Hormone problems can include everything from too little or too much estrogen or testosterone, to associated problems of PMS, perimenopause, menopause, male menopause, and thyroid malfunction.

There are two types of hormone products available: natural and synthetic. Natural hormones are hormones whose molecular structures most closely resemble those made by the body's cells.

Holistic practitioners generally recommend full-body detoxification to remove xenoestrogens first to normalize body functions before resorting to either natural or synthetic hormone therapy. Here are a list of natural products being used in alternative medicine to help correct hormone problems.

- **Wild Yam:** Contains compounds similar to the hormone progesterone.
- **Progesterone Cream:** Contains one or more natural forms of progesterone that can be applied on the skin.
- **Don Quai:** Improves the blood, strengthens the reproductive system, assists the body in using hormones, and is used to treat female problems such as hot flashes, PMS, menopause, and vaginal dryness.
- **Black Cohosh:** Relieves menopausal symptoms, menstrual cramps with back pain, morning sickness, and pain.
- **Blue Cohosh:** Useful for menstrual disorders and nervous disorders.
- **Plant Sterols:** Contain many natural male and female hormone modulators.
- **Ginseng (American, Chinese or Korean):** Strengthens the adrenal and reproductive glands, enhances immune function, stimulates the appetite.
- **Blessed Thistle:** Good for female disorders and increases milk flow in nursing mothers.
- **Yohimbe:** Increases testosterone, libido and blood flow to erectile tissue.
- **Sarsaparilla:** Regulates hormones and is useful for premenstrual syndrome.
- **Damiana:** Used as an aphrodisiac and to remedy sexual and hormonal problems.
- **Melatonin:** Hormone that regulates the pineal gland. Is known to be a free radical scavenger and immune system booster. Helps prevents aging and is also used as an effective sleeping aid.
- **DHEA (Dehydroepiandrosterone):** Is an important base from which key substances, including the hormones testos-

terone, progesterone, and corticosterone can be derived, either directly or indirectly.

● **Saw Palmetto:** Inhibits production of dihydrotestosterone, a form of testosterone that contributes to enlargement of the prostate gland.

Juicing Recipes

The following juicing recipes are a great way to start correcting nutritional deficiencies in your diet. Each one of these drinks is bursting with bio-available vitamins, minerals, enzymes, amino acids, and phytonutrients. If you don't own a quality juicer, you should consider purchasing one. Many health food stores now have juice bars, offering fresh juice conveniently without having to buy your own machine. The main considerations among the top brands are efficiency, the ability to juice continuously, the ability to juice a variety of vegetables including grasses, and ease of clean up. One of the best is the **Green Power Juice Extractor.** This juicer doesn't heat the juice as some do, and ionizes the juice, which no other juicer does. The **Jack Lalane Power Juicer** or the **JuiceMan Juicer** are both good first-time juicers for beginners. If possible, ask the opinion of people who own different machines, perhaps even get a chance to examine or operate one before buying.

The main purpose of juicing is to concentrate nutrients and make them rapidly and easily available to the body. It's best to use 100% organic produce, if available at your local supermarket or health food store. If you don't have access to organic produce, then wash produce well or soak in pure water with about 20 drops of chlorine dioxide (ClO_2) per gallon. Another alternative procedure to remove pesticides, herbicides, and chemicals from the surface of fruits and vegetables is to use old-fashioned Clorox (pure Clorox/hydrochloric acid, not chlorine). Use 1/2 teaspoon per gallon of distilled water. Soak leafy vegetables and berries for

10-15 minutes and root vegetables and heavy-skinned fruits for 15-30 minutes. After Clorox bath, soak in fresh water bath for 5-10 minutes.

Basic Green Drink
4 cups Alfalfa and/or other Sprouts, 4 cups Sunflower and Buckwheat Greens, 1/2 cup Carrot, 1/2 cup sweet Red Pepper, 1/4 cup Parsley, 1 cup Cucumber. Add 1 bunch Wheat Grass (about 3/4" thick), if desired.

Basic Vegetable Juice
5 Carrots, 4 ounces of Spinach, 4 stalks of Celery, 1/2 Red Beet with stem,1 Cucumber (Greens such as Kale, Swiss chard, Bokchoy, Endive, Cabbage, Broccoli and Bell Peppers may be substituted). A little raw Ginger Root, Udo's Choice Oil or 5 Walnuts may be added to taste.

Blood Builder
8 oz. Celery, 3 oz. Cucumber, 2 oz. Parsley, 3 oz. Spinach

Garden Green Drink
4 cups Sprouts, 4 cups Green Tops, 2 cups Kale or Collard Greens, 1 cup Celery

Green Power Cocktail
4 cups Sprouts, 4 cups Green Tops, 1 cup Kale, 1 cup Beet, 1-1/2 cup Wheat Grass

High Vitamin C & E Drink
6 oz. Spinach, 2 oz. Lettuce, 2 oz. Watercress, 4 oz. Carrot, 2 oz. Green Pepper

Insulin Generator
3 oz. Brussels Sprouts, 3-6 oz. Carrot, 3 oz. String Bean, 4 oz. Lettuce

Potassium Special
3 oz. Carrot, 4 oz. Celery, 2 oz. Parsley, 3 oz. Spinach

Skin Cleanse
4 oz. Potato, 4 oz. Celery, 3-6 oz. Carrot, 2 oz. Watercress

Spring Green Drink
4 cups Sprouts, 4 cups Greens, 1-1/2 cups Dandelion Greens, 1-1/4 cups Scallion, 1 cup Carrot

Vegetable/Grass Drink
1-3 oz. Carrot Juice (1-3 carrots), 3 oz. Celery Juice (2 large stalks), 1-1/2 oz. Parsley Juice (5 sprigs), 1-1/2 oz. Wheat Grass. Add other vegetables as desired, e.g., Lettuce, Cucumber. This blend should consist of 80% greens.

Wheat-Beet Juice
1-1/2 oz. Wheat Grass Juice, 1 oz. Beet Juice, 6 oz Cucumber Juice

ACID/ALKALINE FOOD CHART

High Alkaline-Forming Foods	Wheat Grass, Barley Grass, Alfalfa Grass, Kamut Grass, Oat Grass, Spirulina, Chlorella, Spinach, Broccoli, All Sprouts, Kelp, Garlic, Cayenne Pepper, Kombucha Tea.
Mildly Alkaline-Forming Foods	Green Leaf Lettuce, Romaine Lettuce, Peppers (sweet & hot), Cauliflower, Squash, Celery, Cucumber, Onions, Radishes, Watercress, Zucchini, Tomatoes, Carrots, Kale, Eggplant, Parsley, Asparagus, Endive, Chard, Artichokes, Dulse, Red Cabbage, Sweet Potatoes, Yams, Fermented Veggies, Collard Greens, Parsnips, Vegetable Broth, Sea Vegetables, Maitake, Daikon, Shiitake, Reishi, Nori, Umeboshi, Wakame, Ginger Root, Leeks, Red Potatoes, Green Beans, Yellow Beans, Fresh Olives (un-canned without vinegar), Shallots, Dandelion Greens, Edible Flowers, Organic Tea (Green Tea, Ginseng, Bancha, Herbal Tea), Grain Coffee, Stevia, Molasses, Buckwheat, Millet, Brown Rice, Basmati Rice, Lentils, Kidney Beans, Mung Beans, Pinto Beans, Garbanzo Beans, Black-Eyes Peas, Green Peas, Poppy Seeds, Organic Tofu (fermented), Tempeh, Hummus, Apples, Grapes, Raisins, Avocado, Bananas, Dates, Figs, Apricots, Pomegranates, Peaches, Plums, Pears, Rhubarb, Mango, Papaya, Cantaloupe, Oranges, Lemons, Limes, Grapefruit, Cherries, Strawberries, Blueberries, Blackberries, Raspberries, Nectarines, Honeydew, Bee Pollen, Almonds, Almond Butter, Sunflower Seeds, Pumpkin Seeds, Pecans, Macadamia Nuts, Pine Nuts, Sesame Seeds.
Neutral or Slightly Acidic Foods	Wheat, Barley, Kamut, Rye, Spelt, Oats, Amaranth, Buckwheat, Quinoa, Corn, Honey, Most Oils (olive, coconut, flax, borage, sunflower, safflower, sesame, hemp, grape seed), Carob, Organic Butter, Ion-Exchanged Whey, Plain Organic Yogurt, Organic Cottage Cheese, Goat Cheese, Raw Un-pasteurized Milk, Organic Eggs, Salmon, Trout, Free Range Turkey, Organic Chicken Breast, Lamb, Pasta, Apple Cider Vinegar, Tahini, Walnuts, Cashews, Brazil Nuts, Pistachio.

Alkaline Seasonings	Cinnamon, Ginger, Mustard, Chili Pepper, Sea Salt, Miso, Tamari, Curry, Cilantro, Parsnip, Basil, Cumin, Thyme & Most Herbs.
High Alkalizing Minerals	Calcium, Magnesium, Potassium, Sodium, Cesium, Trace Mineral Drops (sea based).
Acid Landmines To Avoid	Pork, Bacon, Ham, Sausage, Pepperoni, Ribs, Shrimp, Clams, Lobster, Scallops, Sardines, Mussels, Oyster, Chicken Wings, Rabbit, Duck, Organ Meats, Processed Cheese, Yogurt (unless 100% organic from a health food store), Coffee, Soda (including all carbonated beverages), Alcohol (beer, liquor), Bottled Fruit Drinks, Sugar, Corn Syrup, High Fructose Corn Syrup, Fructose, Chocolate (cocoa), Candy Bars, Pharmaceutical Drugs, Tobacco/Nicotine, Tap Water, Pesticides, Herbicides, Household Cleaners, Commercial Soap, Shampoo & Cosmetics (must use all natural versions from a health food store), Candy, Cakes, Ice Cream, Pudding, Cookies, Donuts, Jams & Jellies, Yeast and Autolyzed Yeast Extract, Chewing Gum and Breath Mints (unless from a health food store), Aspartame, Nutri-Sweet, Sweet 'N Low, Equal, Sucrose, Artificial Dyes, Artificial Colors, Artificial Flavors, Preservatives, Fluoride (in water & toothpaste), Chlorine, Monosodium Glutamate (MSG), Phosphoric Acid, Sorbic Acid, Stearic Acid, Magnesium Stearate, Glycerin (unless derived from plant sources), Synthetic Vitamins, Inorganic Minerals (as found in most breads, breakfast cereals, packaged foods), Gelatin, Salt (unless purchased in a health food store), Most Canned and Packaged Foods, Breakfast Cereals (unless they're organic without sugar), Microwaved Foods, Irradiated Foods, Fried Foods, Fast Foods, Pasteurized Beverages (Milk, Fruit & Vegetable Juices), Genetically Modified Foods, All Bleached Flours, Bread (unless 100% whole grain, sprouted & organic), Broth & Gravy (from animals), Coffee Creamers, French Fries, Commercial Peanut Butter, Pasta (made from white flour), Hydrogenated or Partially Hydrogenated Fats & Oils, Pickles (unless all natural), Most Condiments (unless organic and all natural) (i.e. ketchup, mustard, mayonnaise, barbeque sauce etc.), chips, crackers, packaged nuts, soy protein concentrate, soy protein isolate.

Footnotes and References:

1. McCabe, Ed, *Oxygen: It's Called The "Breath of God" Because of Its Miraculous Healing Powers!*, Crusador Magazine June-July 2004, Crusador Enterprises, Orlando, FL 2004.
2. McCabe, Ed, *Flood Your Body With Oxygen*, page 47, Energy Publications, Miami, FL, 2003.
3. Young, Dr. Robert, Ph.D., D.Sc., Young, Shelley Redford, L.M.T., *Sick and Tired? Reclaim Your Inner Terrain*, page 58 & opening quote, Woodland Publishing, Pleasant Grove, UT, 2001.
4. Pearson, R.B., *The Dream and Lie of Louis Pasteur*, Sumeria Press, Collingwood, Australia, 1994.
5. Young, Dr. Robert, Ph.D., D.Sc., Young, Shelley Redford, L.M.T., *The pH Miracle*, page 13, Warner Books, Inc. New York, NY, 2002.
6. Fife, Bruce, N.D., *The Detox Book*, page 19, Health Wise Publications, Colorado Springs, CO, 2001.
7. Horowitz, Dr. Leonard, *Healing Celebrations: Miraculous Recoveries Through Ancient Scriptures, Natural Medicine & Modern Science*, page 51, Tetrahedron Publishing Group, Sandpoint, ID, 2000.
8. Kliment, Felicia Drury, *The Acid Alkaline Balance Diet, page 103*, Contemporary Books, New York, NY, 2002.
9. Heart Disease Fact Sheet, Center For Disease Control and Prevention (CDC), http://www.cdc.gov/cvh/library/fs_heart_disease.htm
10. Kliment, Felicia Drury, *The Acid Alkaline Balance Diet,* pages 88 & 89, Contemporary Books, New York, NY, 2002.
11. Khalsa, Karta Purkh S., C.D.-N., R.H., *Body Balance: Vitalize Your Health With pH Power*, pages 224 & 225, Kensington Publishing Corp., New York, NY, 2004.

Bibliography:

1. Vasey, Christopher, N.D., *The Acid – Alkaline Diet for Optimum Health*, Healing Arts Press, Rochester, VT, 2003.
2. Baroody, Theodore A., *Alkalize or Die,* Holographic Health, Waynesville, NC, 1991.
3. Béchamp, Pierre Jacques Antoine, *The Blood and Its Third Anatomical Element*, John Ouseley LTD., London, England, 1912.
4. Enderlein, Prof. Dr. Günther, *Akmon,* Vol. I, Book 2, Hamburg, Germany: Ibica-Verlarg, 1957.
5. Hume, E. Douglas, *Béchamp or Pasteur? A Lost Chapter in the History of Biology,* 1st ed. Ashingdon, Rochford, Essex, England: The C.W. Daniel Company, 1923; 2d. ed. (London: C.W. Daniel

Company, 1932) reprinted by Health Research, Pomeroy, WA, 1989.

6. Livingston-Wheeler, Virginia, M.D., *The Conquest of Cancer,* Franklin Watts, New York, 1984.
7. Bleker, Dr. Maria, *Blood Examination in Darkfield according to Prof. Dr. Günther Enderlein,* Semmelweis-Verlag, Gesamtherstellung, Germany, 1993.
8. Meyerowitz, Steve, *Wheat Grass – Nature's Finest Medicine,* Sproutman Publications, Great Barrington, MA, 1998.
9. Rapp, Doris J., M.D., *Our Toxic World,* Personal Transformation Press, Penryn, CA, 2003.
10. Costantini, A.V., Weiland, H., Qvick, Lars I., *The Fungal/Mycotoxin Etiology of Human Disease,* Vol. 1&2, Johann Friedrich Oberlin Verlag, Freiburg, Germany, 1994.
11. Erasmus, Udo, *Fats that Heal, Fats that Kill,* Alive Books, Burnaby, B.C., Canada, 1993.
12. Clark, Hulda, Ph.D., N.D., *The Cure For All Cancers,* New Century Press, Chula Vista, CA, 1993.
13. Clark, Hulda, Ph.D., N.D., *The Cure For All Diseases,* New Century Press, Chula Vista, CA, 1995.
14. Goldberg, Burton, *Alternative Medicine, The Definitive Guide,* Celestial Arts, Berkeley, CA, 2002.
15. Balch, Phyllis A., CNC, *Prescription For Nutritional Healing, The A-Z Guide To Supplements,* Avery, New York, NY, 2002.
16. Balch, Phyllis A., CNC, *Prescription For Nutritional Healing, Third Edition,* Avery, New York, NY, 2000.
17. Balch, Phyllis A., CNC, *Prescription For Herbal Healing, An Easy-to-Use A-to-Z Reference to Hundreds of Common Disorders and Their Herbal Remedies,* Avery, New York, NY, 2002.
18. Mercola, Dr. Joseph, *Total Health Cookbook & Program,* Mercola.com, Schaumburg, IL, 2004.
19. Appleton, Nancy, Ph.D., *The Curse of Louis Pasteur,* Choice Publishing, Santa Monica, CA, 1999.
20. Appleton, Nancy, Ph.D., *Lick The Sugar Habit,* Avery, New York, NY, 1996.

Glossary

Aerobic: Requiring air or free oxygen for life; pertaining to or caused by the presence of oxygen.

Allopathic: Conventional western medicine. The method of treating disease by the use of agents (drugs), producing effects different or opposite from those of the disease treated. (Allopathic physicians treat disease symptoms instead of disease causes.)

Anaerobic: Living in the absence of air or free oxygen; pertaining to or caused by the absence of oxygen.

ATP: Adenosine triphosphate, an ester of adenosine and triphosphoric acid, serving as a source of energy for physiological reactions, especially muscle contraction.

Autogenesis: Self produced; self generated. Pertaining to substances or processes generated in the body.

Autoimmune Disease: A disease of the immune system where the defenses turn against the body itself. This leads to chronic and often deadly diseases. Many researchers believe that in some cases a virus infection may "retain" the body's defense cells to attack the wrong tissues. Many of these diseases have periods of crisis and periods of no symptoms.

Cell Asphyxiation: A state in which the body's cells choke, suffocate, smother, or die. Can be caused by a number of internal and external factors such as: lack of oxygen, poor circulation, lack of cellular nutrition, too many toxins built up within and around the cell.

Cellular Terrain: The ecological environment within the cell and the condition of the fluids that surround the cell.

Congestive Toxicosis: An unnatural accumulation of toxins in an organ or part.

Cytopathy: The study of cellular disease.

Dark-field Microscopy: A special microscope technology that uses scattered light, with the object set against a dark background (field). It allows viewing of much smaller particles than an ordinary instrument.

Degenerative Disease: Any disease in which there is decay of structure or function of tissue. Some kinds of degenerative disease are arteriosclerosis, osteoarthritis.

Epidemiology: The study of the spread, prevention, and control of disease.

Flora: A colony of bacteria and other microorganisms that grow normally in the intestines without which we could not remain in good health. There are 10 times more bacteria in the digestive system than there are cells in the entire body. There are more than 400 species of bacteria found in the digestive system. These include both beneficial and harmful species, which continually compete to maintain a well-balanced intestinal flora.

Free Radical: An atom or compound in which there is an unpaired electron. A free radical reacts quickly with other molecules. Despite what we've been led to believe a free radical can be either good or bad. Oxygen, which is a free radical, is needed by the body for life. The immune system creates oxygen based free radicals to bond with and neutralize toxic compounds in the body. A free radical that enters the body as a result of exposure to toxic substances from food, air, water, vaccines, etc. becomes harmful when there's not enough oxygen to bond to it and rid it from the body. These renegade toxic free radicals can damage DNA and cells.

Herxheimer Reaction: An increase in symptoms after a drug is given. The reaction was first seen in penicillin treatment of syphilis, but has been found to occur in other diseases as well. This term is often used in alternative medicine to describe a condition that occurs when the body detoxifies too quickly.

Homeopathy (homeopathic): A system of healing based on the theory that "like cures like." The theory was advanced in the late eighteen century by Dr. Samuel Hahnemann who believed that very small doses of medicine could produce particular symptoms of disease, thus triggering the immune system to combat the disease naturally. In essence, homeopathic medicine jump starts your immune system to target a specific health condition.

Homeostasis: The physiological process by which the internal systems of the body (e.g. blood pressure, body temperature, acid-base balance) are maintained at equilibrium, despite variations in the external conditions.

Hypoxia: Too little oxygen in the cells. Symptoms include turning blue, too fast a heart rate, high blood pressure, contractions of blood vessels, dizziness, and mental confusion. The tissues most sensitive to hypoxia are the brain, heart, vessels of the lungs, and liver.

Immuno-Suppressed: A condition where the body's resistance to infection and other foreign bodies is suppressed. When the body is in an "immuno-suppressed" state, it is much more susceptible to infection and certain types of cancer.

Metabolic Disease: A disease condition pertaining to, or affected by metabolism. A disorder that interferes with normal digestion and use of food in the body.

Metastasis: The distant spread of a malignant tumor from its site of origin. This occurs by three main routes: (1) through the bloodstream; (2) through the lymphatic system; (3) across body cavities.

Microorganism: A tiny animal or plant able to carry on living processes. Kinds of microorganisms include bacteria, viruses, parasites, fungi, protozoa.

Microzymas: Tiny indestructible living enzymes present in all cells and bodily fluids capable of multiplying. Microzymas also transmit signals to cells to replicate life. When cells become diseased microzymas will transmit signals to trigger a fermentation process to bring an organism back to the dust of the ground unless health is re-established.

Mitochondria: A small, threadlike organ within the cytoplasm of a cell that controls cell life and breathing. Mitochondria are the main source of cell energy.

Modulate: To regulate by or adjust to a certain measure or proportion. To attune to a certain pitch or key. Used in reference to the immune system; immune system modulation.

Monomorphism: Having only form. Used in reference to Louis Pasteur's Germ Theory of Disease where he believed outside invasion of germs was the sole cause of disease.

Morbid Microforms: A term used to describe unwanted and unhealthy bacteria, viruses, parasites, fungi, etc. that are involved in the disease process.

Mutation: The act or process of changing or altering in a person's genes that occurs by itself with or without the influence of a mutagen. Genes are stable units, but a mutation often is passed on to future generations.

Mycotoxin: A waste product from yeast or fungus.

Naturopathy (naturopathic): A method of treating disease using food, nutrition, sunshine, fresh air, massage, detoxification, exercise, heat, etc., to assist the natural healing process.

Paradigm Shift: In 1962, Thomas Kuhn wrote The Structure of Scientific Revolution, and fathered, defined and popularized the concept of "paradigm shift" (p.10). Kuhn argues that scientific advancement is not evolutionary, but rather is a "series of peaceful interludes punctuated by intellectually violent revolutions," and in those revolutions "one conceptual world view is replaced by another." Think of a Paradigm shift as a change from one way of thinking to another. It's a revolution, a transformation, a sort of metamorphosis. It just does not happen, but rather it is driven by agents of change.

pH: Acronym for the power of hydrogen and used as a symbol to determine the level of acidity or alkalinity of a solution.

Pleomorphism (pleomorphic): The rapid change of both form and function of a microform during a life cycle (i.e. bacteria to virus, virus to parasite, parasite to fungus, etc.)

Systemic Disease: A disease condition that affects the whole body rather than a single area or part of the body.

Toxemia: The presence of poisons (toxins) from bacteria in the body's tissues, cells, and blood.

For a **free** catalog of books and booklets published and distributed by CRUSADOR ENTERPRISES Call 1-800-593-6273 or send the completed form to the address below, or fax it to 1-407-297-4094

Crusador Enterprises
P.O. Box 618205
Orlando, FL 32861-8205

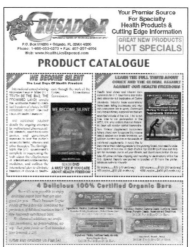

Please send me a FREE catalog!

FIRST NAME _____

LAST NAME _____

COMPANY (IF APPLICABLE) _____

MAILING ADDRESS _____

CITY _____ STATE _____ ZIP _____

PHONE (___) _____

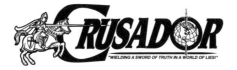

www.HealthTruthRevealed.com

ORDER BULK COPIES OF THE #1 HEALTH BOOK ON THE MARKET

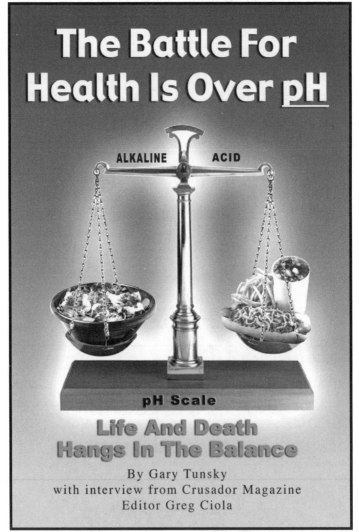

If you've found this book extremely informative and you'd like to help spread the truth, order bulk copies to pass out to everone you know. Call **1-800-593-6273** for discount rates.

Sign Up To Receive CRUSADOR's Weekly E-alerts FREE!

STAY CURRENT ON ALL THE LATEST NEWS!

CRUSADOR E-alerts bring you current, hard-hitting news on many very important breaking health issues. So much is happening on a daily basis that it's physically impossible through our printed publication to keep our readers fully informed. *CRUSADOR E-alerts* are a great opportunity for us to bond with our readers and communicate with them on a much more frequent basis. Instead of you having to go online to do the hard research to stay informed, we'll do the hard work for you. Once a week you'll open your e-mail to some of the most powerful health stories you'll find anywhere. The best part of all is that we're offering this wonderful service FREE of charge. Just log on to **www.HealthTruthRevealed.com** and register your e-mail address and you're in. So don't delay – sign up today!

Some of the topics we cover:

- **Genetic Engineering**
- **Pharmaceutical Dangers**
- **Vaccines**
- **Food Toxins**
- **Health Lies Exposed**
- **Cancer Myths**
- **Alternative Medicines**
- **Healthy Alternatives**
- **And much more...**

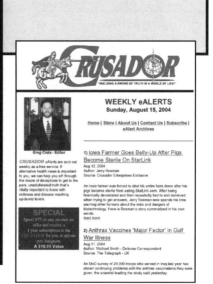

www.HealthTruthRevealed.com

Subscribe To *CRUSADOR*

If you'd like to stay informed on a number of very important health issues, you need to subscribe to *CRUSADOR*. With sickness and disease running rampant, you and your loved ones need a reputable source for health truth. In a world of half-truths and outright lies, you can't afford to be without this vital information – the stakes are too high. You can order a one-year subscription (6-issues) for $20.00 or a two-year subscription (12-issues) for just $35.00. To sign up today call **1-800-593-6273** or visit our website at: **www.HealthTruthRevealed.com**. Here are just a few of the topics the newsletter covers in great detail.

- The Latest In Alternative Medicine
- Dangerous Toxins Hidden In Your Foods
- Cancer Myths
- The Dangers Of Mercury
- The Ongoing Genetic Engineering Debacle
- The Corporate Takeover Of America's Farms
- The Harmful Dangers Of Pharmaceutical Drugs
- The Toxic Effects Of Vaccines
- The Environmental Impact Of Pesticides, Herbicides, and Fertilizer

Thank you
Antoine Béchamp

Your memory,
hard work,
and scientific discoveries
have not been forgotten!